Instructions not included

One Mum, Three Boys and a Very
Steep Learning Curve

Charlotte Moerman

1 3 5 7 9 10 8 6 4 2

Virgin Books, an imprint of Ebury Publishing,
20 Vauxhall Bridge Road,
London SW1V 2SA

Virgin Books is part of the Penguin Random House group of companies
whose addresses can be found at global.penguinrandomhouse.com

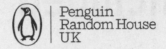

Penguin
Random House
UK

First published in the United Kingdom by Virgin Books in 2009

www.penguin.co.uk

A CIP catalogue record for this book is available from the British Library

ISBN 9780753553831

Printed and bound in Great Britain by Clays Ltd, Elcograf S.p.A.

Penguin Random House is committed to a sustainable future for our
business, our readers and our planet. This book is made from Forest
Stewardship Council® certified paper.

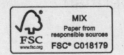

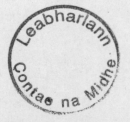

For Bram and the boys, of course

Acknowledgements

Heartfelt thanks to all those who mopped my brow, drip-fed encouragement and endured my continual blathering during the writing of this book.

Thanks to Bram for keeping all the balls in the air while I installed myself at the PC. For minding the boys, for consenting to being sent up, for bolstering me along the way, and for being there far more often than he is given credit.

Thank you also to the boys for taking it on the chin and for their unfailing enthusiasm: 'Mummy, is that your book? It looks *really* good.' And for telling anyone who cared to ask that 'Mummy makes us sit outside while she is writing'.

Thanks to my mum, Lynne, for her enduring feedback, love and support. And to my dad, Ray, for maintaining his belief in me, even though he says I haven't portrayed him grumpily enough.

Thanks to Catherine Hanly at Raising Kids for giving me my blogging break. To Patrick Walsh at Conville and Walsh for seeing potential in the blog and encouraging me whole-heartedly to give it a go. And to Louisa Joyner and Mary Instone at Virgin Books for their guidance and advice, and for making the process of turning my story into a book such good fun.

Thanks to Avril and Caroline, and to Sarah, Ema and Gemma for geeing me along just when I needed it. To Thomas, Maisy, Charlie and Lola *et al* for furnishing me with some Really Useful ideas along the way. And to all my friends and family for providing the inspiration for this book.

Prologue

It's early Sunday evening. We're on the sofa. Storm-damaged cushions lie crushed under three pairs of shifting pyjama-clad buttocks and my own more heavily anchored ones. My other half and *his* besuited buttocks are making their way to Islamabad. It's just me, our three boys and an ill-judged cup of coffee.

Once the cushions were blue, now they're a sort of bilge. Spilt milk, furtively wiped snot and the odd little accident before bedtime have all taken their toll. I've no idea how, but I could swear that every time I come back into the room the stains seem to have mated.

I occasionally wonder if I might give that Tracey woman a run for her money. How do you get nominated for a shot at the Turner Prize anyway? I'm thinking this could be a real knock-out: *My Sofa* – an installation, consisting of our own dirty and defeated sofa, strewn with used tissues, partly decomposed rice cakes and a couple of leaky felt-tips. Scrawled around the walls would be a list of *Everyone Who Has Ever Trampled Here with Their Shoes On 2002–2008*.

Sometimes I feel I'm not unlike the sofa. I try my best to be bright and fresh and useful. And I must've looked OK at one time because someone chose me. These days though, I often feel a bit sat upon, I'm sagging in places where I shouldn't and frankly I'm a bit tired, a bit muted but not in a Farrow & Ball stylish kind of way.

I have spent the last five minutes blotting at the armrest with an Aloe Vera baby wipe, wondering who this much-greeted Vera is anyway. The boys had had a disagreement over whose was the comic they were poring over, which led to a shove and a shout and a stray elbow causing warm coffee to seep into my jeans and the arm of the beleaguered sofa. The tussle was over in an instant and the boys fell swiftly silent. I gulped back my wrath, staunched the tears that nearly followed and reached for the eternally handy pack of Pampers wipes. How did I ever live without them?

Dirk left for Heathrow an hour ago. Sunday departures are the worst. Weekends are family time by rights, but our weekends are often interrupted by the distant call of a tannoyed flight announcement. 'This is the last and final call for passenger Moerman on Flight BA 521 to Somewhere Else. Please make your way to your gate immediately where the cabin crew will be happy to welcome you on board with a newspaper and refreshments of your choice. Please note that in the interests of passenger comfort, namely yours, all family baggage will have been offloaded and left behind at home with your wife. May I take this opportunity to wish you a very pleasant flight?'

He'll be away until Friday. Before he went, he kissed the boys, asked them to look after Mummy and gave me a peck on the cheek whilst grabbing his codjecar. Don't be mistaken into thinking my other half is a sad middle-aged bloke pretending to be a crotch-clutching rap artist. I can't see him with a gold front tooth or sporting that low-slung-trousers flash-your-pants look. That said, perhaps he *could* rebrand himself as Disappear in a Puff of Pink Smoke Daddy.

Because he *does* disappear quite a lot, our Puff, taking his battered passport with him. He slips into the taxi and closes the door on his bleary-eyed wife, our flotsam and jetsam of house contents, and the knot of small boys all bleating 'The batteries have run out Daddy'. And then, in the blink of an indicator, he's gone.

Codjecar, to remove any doubt, is the term used universally in our house for the trolley-dolly suitcase that accompanies our main, well, *only* breadwinner, on his globetrotting business travels. It's one of those toddler-invented words that struck you as kind of cute, so you decide to keep and use it. Sometimes in the presence of non-family, too. It's a measure of just how addled you become as a parent when all of a sudden you think it's acceptable to use words like 'codjecar', 'mamalamouche' and 'cocklit' in company.

I bung the browned wipes into the kitchen bin and return to the living room as the phone starts to ring. Billy's switching on the telly, my peace offering and a bedtime treat for all. The ever-ebullient Pui bursts onto the screen with Chris who today is playing a glockenspiel. I wonder what the difference is between a glockenspiel and a xylophone. I wonder if I should be worried that I instinctively wish that Chris would turn to Pui and clonk her on the head with his glockenspiel stick. I wonder if I'm going to get to the phone before it rings off.

'Hello?'

'Hi there. It's me.'

'Hi, me. Got there OK?'

'Slow traffic but I'm in the lounge now, boarding in five minutes. Boys OK?'

'Fine. Sofa's less happy though.'

'Sofa?'

'Just a little spillage. Want to say goodnight to Daddy, boys?'

'Mmnph.'

'I *said* does anyone want to say goodnight to Daddy?'

'Good-er-night, Daddy!' (Sid, with his customary extra syllable for luck.)

'Goodnight, then. Go get your plane.'

'Goodnight. Love you.'

The phone clicks into silence.

The boys, unphased, are watching a repeat of Catherine Tate reading a CBeebies *Bedtime Hour* story called 'Krong'. None of it's weird to them: a time traveller reading them a story about aliens in their own living room. Sometimes here in a comfy chair, sometimes there in a deceptively spacious Police Box. Sometimes doing funny voices, sometimes playing it straight. Not unlike Daddy, who's sometimes here and sometimes there. Or, more accurately, often there and not so often here.

Are they bovvered? Not at this particular moment it seems. Am I bovvered? I slink in beside my clean-smelling, damp-haired brood and pull the nearest one onto my lap.

'I love you, Mummy,' whispers Jack.

'I love you too,' I murmur. 'We'll be OK,' I add, before realising I'm leaning against the wet patch and shifting myself along a little.

Chapter 1

We're in the kitchen. Soup is simmering gently on the stove. The microwave beep-beep-beep-beeps. Dirk squeezes my shoulder. 'This is it then. Over the top.' I know this isn't the most significant part of my pregnancy. And I know I shouldn't be nervous. But Dirk's effervescent high spirits are giving me the jitters. I grab the wooden spoon and give the soup a vigorous stir. Hot liquid spatters over the side and fizzes angrily into the gas flame. There'll be black streaks on the underside of the pan to tackle later on. The trouble is, the more I procrastinate, the bigger the mess I seem to be making.

There's a fish pie browning in the oven. It's been there for quite some time and smells promising. I take a peek through the seventies-style sunglass-brown oven door and am reassured at the sight of the nicely bubbling cheese topping. Of course it will leave a ring of encrusted dregs that, like the saucepan, will need a thorough scrubbing later on. But you can't have your (fish) cake and eat it, so for now at least I blank that bit out.

Dirk's gone off to the other room, gassing with my parents. It's evening. Everyone bar me seems relaxed. I glance around the chaotic kitchen: a measuring jug, a debris-strewn chopping board and a clutch of knives lie willy-nilly across the surfaces. My cooking style's a little muddled at the best of times, but if I keep my fingers crossed it usually turns out all right on the night. Unless I try to do something a bit clever, in which case disaster looms. Tonight, though, the fruit of my labours in the kitchen is the least of my concerns. There are bigger fish to fry.

It's Christmas Eve, a night of great expectations. There's a huge Nordic Spruce shimmering in the corner of the room. Its branches are weighed down with both Sally Ann trinkets from the early Christmases of our marriage and more recent baubles picked up locally. The former charity shop trophies are naturally, to me, worth a thousand of the latter. I know better than to let this on to Dirk, having spent a small fortune going to town on this year's tree. ''Tis the season to spend loads of lolly ... fa la la la laaa, la la la lah!'

This is our first Christmas in Highbury and in my usual understated way I've gone completely overboard. There are tastefully wrapped gifts piled extravagantly high under the tree, upmarket 'luxury gift' crackers and a full complement of white fairy lights, most of them working too. There are candles, of course, a bit of holly, and a strategically placed sprig of mistletoe that's got Dad's eyes twinkling like the lights adorning the tree.

We've also dragged out the faded red stocking that mum made for me as a child. The embroidery thread spelling out my name is a little jaded and cotton wool is coming off in clumps at the top. But Christmas just wouldn't be Christmas without it. Twenty-eight-year-olds *will* be twenty-eight-year-olds, eh? Who needs youngsters to make Christmas magical when you've big kids like me and Dad around to fill in the gap?

Christmas would never be the same again.

A few years hence and the tree is no longer colour-coordinated, there are festive steam trains and robots hanging from its boughs and the lights absolutely must flash. Multicoloured is good. We've got a chocolate Advent calendar ('When is it *my* turn?'), a whole row of expectant stockings and the greenery has been replaced with tinsel. Some days I wonder if I've been transported down the Nags Head when I take in the gaudy fronds across the mantelpiece and twined around the pictures as tasteful as Marlene's dress sense and almost as loud as her laugh.

The pile of gifts of course, is still ludicrously mountainous, though the paper's all grinning polar bears and penguins in woolly scarves. I still spend the run-up to Christmas spending but in a different way. I pride myself on being a mean hunter-gatherer of 3-for-2 and BOGOF offers, and I am particularly precious about my sale-bargain present drawer. It is my defence against the creeping guilt of frittering away another twenty pounds here and there on more new toys when we already have a houseful anyway. Money that I have not earned. I am now without income of any sort; I am the Queen of Guilty Outgoings.

And then I stroke down the hair of my sleeping boys and I don't give a toss about the bank balance for at least ten minutes.

For them, I would love to recreate the Christmases of my own childhood: rosy-cheeked, magical. There would be the thrill of nudging the bulging stocking at the edge of the duvet in the morning, the promise of a new Sindy Doll or the long-awaited Mouse Trap game and, before any of that, what could be better than a festive breakfast of Mum's scrambled eggs, cooked slowly, ever so slowly, to moist perfection and served on meltingly hot buttered toast? Sheer happiness on a plate.

I'd love to cook scrambled eggs on toast for my lot at Christmas, or any time, really. But they don't do scrambled eggs. They don't do toast made from the organic honey and sunflower bread I've got in the cupboard. And they're not terribly keen on butter either.

7

Not sure where I went wrong. I bought the Annabel Karmel book that promised to 'encourage diversity' and 'consolidate good eating habits'. I shopped at Fresh and Wild for the fruit and veg that I lovingly pureed and dolloped into ice-cube trays which had never had it so good. And I even chose a really special melamine dinner set to feed them off, complete with a smart blue tractor, a shiny yellow dumper truck and a forklift, its driver inexplicably hefting off a worried-looking cow.

Perhaps that was the problem. How could they pay attention to the hard-hatted workman in the middle of the plate with his encouraging 'Go' sign when their sensibilities were being offended by the sight of a cow on her way to the abattoir? Especially given the driver is sporting what can only be described as a maniacal grin. Goodness, it's enough to put anyone off their pureed beef gloop. Hard Hat man might have just as well held up a 'Stop' sign and had done with it.

But Christmas lunches would be different, I always felt. OK, so scrambled eggs and ground beef remain 'off' for a while, but surely a steaming plate of turkey with all the trimmings would go down swimmingly. Surely it would all be wolfed down in a scene of domestic bliss.

I would be Lynda Bellingham, pouring gravy over the spuds. Dirk would be the dad, making festive leg and breast jokes whilst sharpening the carving knife. And the boys would sit rosy-faced and obedient at table, paper crowns atop their heads, turkey being appreciatively put away by hearty young appetites.

Instead we have a set of reluctant diners, guilty streaks of chocolate still smeared around their mouths, self-aware young urbanites who really don't want to wear *those* on their heads and half-empty Tyrell Katz plates with a lone chipolata, a couple of token carrots and the bargaining chip blob of ketchup at the side.

It always makes me so pleased to have queued outside the butchers for my free-range, additive-free, but sadly not *free* turkey. Still, at least I get a measure of satisfaction splodging ketchup over Hard Hat man.

We're all sitting down at the dining room table, a 2+2 parody of Christmas meals of yore when it was my parents, my brother Ed and me. I'm as quiet as a church mouse. Dirk looks like the cat that got the cream. The steam from the soup flushes my cheeks. Dirk tops up the glasses, all but mine. My parents detect something fishy.

'What's there to be nervous about?' asked Dirk as I'd cut up the salmon earlier in the day. He encircled his arms around me from behind as he spoke, a move he's perfected with martial art precision: I pull a sharp knife out of the utensils drawer, ready to dice or slice, and nine times out of ten he moves in for a quick spoon on spoon hug. And then he starts to tickle. I thought all kids were taught not to run with scissors. Perhaps we should ensure that not tickling with knives is slipped into the syllabus too?

I shrugged him off, but I knew he was right. This should be one of the most exciting announcements of my life. I was neither in my teens, unmarried, nor about to expose a whoops-here-comes-a-baby, torrid affair. No big dramarama. So why the collywobbles?

'I don't know. I just feel something heavy in the pit of my stomach.'

'Oven. Bun in. Rearrange.'

I glowered at him over my shoulder.

'It's just ...' I put down the knife and laid it next to the cold, slippery orange flesh on the chopping board.

It's just ... what? The uncertainty of divulging all whilst still only nine weeks gone? All the books say wait till twelve and I'm not a rule-breaker by habit. The end of the bubble of *just us*. The terribly British embarrassment about admitting we'd ... shh ... had sex (seven years of marriage and that's a heck of a way of converting the itch)? The bad manners of preceding my elder sibling onto the parental starting blocks, especially when I know they've been trying? The fear of what I'll be leaving behind? The fear of the changes ahead? The fear of the unknown? Or the fear that voicing it'd make becoming a mum more terrifyingly real?

'I don't really know,' I said again, verbalising none of my skittering doubts. For a girl with a degree, a Pitman Training Basic Computer Skills diploma and a Cycling Proficiency certificate, I seemed at that moment to not know an awful lot. (Including how to handle split infinitives.)

Denying any further eye contact, I picked up the knife and continued to jab petulantly at the fish in a, to me, particularly satisfying way. To Dirk I must have been quite exasperating. I took no notice. It was going to be no picnic being pregnant and giving birth at the end of all this, not to mention what lay in the murky world thereafter.

Dirk took the hint and left the room. He's good at that, I thought, leaving.

He seems to be taking things in his stride, of course, my husband. While I, typically, am making a meal of things. He doesn't seem perturbed by the big change that's about to happen. That is already happening. My body and my life are already changing irreparably. And there's plenty more to come. Sure, he'll be as involved as he possibly can be. But still, there's no getting away from the fact that, unless something freakily tabloid-fodder has gone on, the male half of the equation does not and cannot experience all the trimmings.

The father of an impending child will not develop a pea-sized bladder overnight and a tonne-weight intrusion pressing onto it in the wee small hours. He will not get sudden heartburn, stretch marks or the threat (and that alone is enough to have anyone running scared) of an episiotomy. He does not do labour. Or transform into a dairy cow. He does not have to sneeze sitting down for the rest of his life if he stuffs up the Pelvic Floor Exercises. He does not have to morph into a new and unknown version of himself. Or agree to spend the foreseeable future with a new constant companion that he hasn't been able to pre-select from the Internet. He does not have to do any of these things. Or if he does, he must be a pretty unique individual and Max Clifford will ensure that he gets paid handsomely for it.

Make no bones, I am over overjoyed at being pregnant. It's not the immediate changes to my body that are worrying me either. I don't particularly mind about those, they are all part of the journey, and I am determined to remain master of my own pelvic floor with plenty of early below-the-belt workouts. It is just that I feel a bit baffled about the future. And who it is that I will be sharing it with.

'So, what's all this about then, Chaz?' intones Dad, ever the softly-softly subtle kind of guy. Mum's eyes are saucer-wide. I pause and then a grin erupts on my face like I've just had a mouthful of Space Dust.

'Well, I guess it's time to let the cat out of the bag. You've probably already twigged and, um, I'm not sure how to say this but ... you're (coughs) going to be grandparents.'

'Ooh,' squeals Mum impulsively, probably wondering why I'd been rambling on to her earlier about inconsequentials like where I'd bought my Brussels this year, or how I planned to cook the roast potatoes. I wonder why I did, too.

Everyone is all broad smiles and glinting eyes. The glow from the Christmas tree now seems comparatively dull. Flushed cheeks, astonished congratulations and spontaneous hugs take centre stage as the spot swings firmly to this end of the room. I feel sheepish after behaving so badly earlier. Everyone is now treating me like a star. I am sitting in my dressing room before a mirror framed in lights, adoring fans flocking to my door with flowers, cards and underpants, just as if I were Tom Jones. I love the reassuring attention, and the pants might come in handy too, now that I'll be going up a size or two.

'Well, well, well!' says Dirk to cover up the gush whilst producing the obligatory bottle of bubbly. Well trained in his humour, I instinctively picture three holes in the ground. I feel bad about shutting him out earlier. This pregnancy's a shared journey. He's probably just as scared as me. I'd better stop thinking of myself as the VIP in greasepaint and remember that this one is a double act. Who are we anyway, I wonder, Morcambe and Wise? Cannon and Ball? The Two Ronnies?

There's a resounding pop, the fizz of champagne and we all toast the impending birth of Christ and/or our first (grand)child in no particular order.

'So it's "Cheers" from me.'

'And it's "Cheers" from him.'

'Cheers!'

Once the dust settles, we get on with it. Christmas I mean. And nurturing our baby. Mum keeps giving me twinkly-eyed grins. Dad keeps mentioning the brick wall knowingly.

Having children, Dad has said for as long as I can remember, is the equivalent of having a six-foot edifice of bricks and mortar spring suddenly into your life. To be honest, I'm not really sure what he means. It's just a standing joke that 1+1=3 and a large brick wall. Perhaps it's that life, as you've always known it, slams to a sudden halt in your face. Perhaps it's something like, OK, so far you've been concentrating on the foundations, now let the real work begin. Or perhaps it's just a clever crossword clue that I'm too dim to work out. Dunno. Some things you're just not meant to understand. Like why are blueberries black, like why are clowns so *creepy*, like what on earth's the 'Ning Nang Nong' poem all about. You just accept these things for what they are and enjoy them. OK, well maybe not the clown with the trousers that keep falling down. He's for specialist tastes.

Talking of cows that go bong, if I were to cast an actor to play my dad in a film, Spike Milligan would be an excellent choice. Just like Spike, Dad's a genius of a man but he's also quite unfathomable at times. Only of course the Goon is no more, so I'll have to find someone else. Jack Nicholson, perhaps? Yes, I think I'm onto something there. It's all in the eyebrows.

He's all right, my dad. I'd give him Best Supporting Dad Oscar any day: 'Great Supporting Dads have a magical power to transport us to a different time and place. And so, for his unique but sometimes baffling phraseology; for his bottomless knowledge on birds and wild flowers, Bull and Bear markets, Dave Brubeck and King Edward spuds; for his matchless approach to DIY; for his ongoing inventions and projects that one of these days will make him a Del Boy millionaire; for his ability to talk to anyone about anything; and for his palpable devotion and unfailing confidence in his little girl grown big, I give you, My Dad.' (Wild applause.)

Mum is much more of an open book. And this is no bad thing. She should by rights be played by Marilyn, except that Marilyn, like Spike, has taken her Equity Card to the great casting couch in the sky. So perhaps Julie Christie then? A classic English Rose, tick. Ice-blue eyes, tick. Rapunzel-like blonde hair, oh yes, she'd be just perfect. And then there's her longevity too. She's refused to hang up her fur hat ahead of time. She's dug her heels in, stayed the distance and blimey doesn't she wear it well? Plus, of course, she's used to spending time with guys with eyebrows so I'd say she's made for the job. Sign her up immediately.

Women are complicated. Daughters and mothers are complicated. But I can genuinely say that our lives have been a lot less complicated than an epic David Lean drama-romance-war film. Hand on heart, we seem to have rubbed along OK all these years and she's not yet taken up her customer right to return me – product damaged, faulty or not lived up to expectations; statutory rights not affected; postage paid at destination under terms of contract – in a brown paper parcel back to the shop.

We've shared a lot: puddings, shoes and hotel beds. Shopping sprees. Diets. Revision sessions: me my GSCEs, she her mature student finals at Cambridge. She took me to my first bra-fitting; she took me to my wedding-dress-fitting. She took me to my first ever concert (Paul Simon, *Graceland* tour) and she took me on a couple of girls-only holidays including a memorable cycling trip around a clutch of medieval hilltop villages in France. As I panted my way towards the promised *village fleuri*, all ramparts and restaurants and 429 flipping metres above sea level, I gritted my teeth and hummed 'You Can Call Me Al' again and again to myself for comfort. I wondered if, on this occasion, perhaps mother didn't always know best.

You can bet that my faith was restored, though, when we got to the top of the hill and the Lion D'Or, its vine-covered alfresco terrace and hand-chalked blackboard menu beckoning us enticingly to its door. This was the time we shared out first taste of garlic-buttered frogs' legs together. And as the sun went down over the magnificent view I realised I was no longer hopping mad about the tortuous ascent.

• • •

I will never of course be able to replicate a girls-only holiday in my own capacity as mum. Unless I leave all the boys somewhere and bugger off alone. Appealing thought on some days, I must confess.

We do, as it happens, manage an experimental week one summer with the family splitting off in different directions. Only it's not me that's on my tod. The boys and I stay a second holiday week in Suffolk while Dirk hurtles back to London for work. And while he's gone back to Mind the Gap, my parents have come along to fill the one he's left. I manage alone a lot of the time, but on holiday I want more than the company of under-fives, thank you very much. This is the life, I think.

'Sometimes it's hard to think of what life was like before them,' says Mum.

'You can say that again.'

'Do you think you'll have any more?'

'Oh, I don't think so. It kills me to say it, but three's enough. Don't you think?'

'Then you'll need to start thinking about what you'll be doing next, then.'

'Yes, Mum,' I nod, smiling in spite of myself, feeling twelve all over again.

'You can't put it off for ever you know.'

When I hopped it from the nest and went and got married, of course my relationship with Mum changed. So, my prince came along and give me a smackeroo and I transformed into, well, the grown-up me. And I'm very happy being the grown-up me, thank you very much. But still, it's nice to go back and hang out in the company of my mum. I feel completely at ease with her. I am me, not needing to hide or create smokescreens. We can luxuriate in being unutterably ourselves and happily fritter away time together.

I can't recall ever having kept any secrets from her. Well, OK, when I was a child I might have binned the half-full Um Bongo carton from my Snoopy lunchbox, gradually and concertedly picked off the previous inhabitant's *Wacky Races* wallpaper from inside my bedroom cupboard, and nurtured a fledgling admiration for the rebellious and much-peroxided Bo Duke. I was quite clearly a wild child.

When I grew up though, I realised Bo wouldn't have me, and that I probably didn't want him either. (I wonder what ever happened to him, that cool red General Lee car and Daisy Duke's very short shorts?) I had my very own Bo with a much better grasp of the Highway Code. Mum was always there at the other end of the phone and we had regular chinwags. We chat a lot. We are like the ancient hanging gardens. We tend to Babylon.

So with a track record of keeping, well, little of any substance from the auspices of my mum, it had been a bit odd to hide such an earth-shattering secret from her. Especially those times when I'd felt a little unsteady, a tad nauseous and not a little like a novice cyclist: a bit shaky and afraid of falling off.

Ill, low or just plain scared – as in the case of my frantic visit to the hospital's Early Pregnancy Unit, seven weeks and spotting – I'd usually be straight on the blower to share and dilute my angst. With Mum. Dirk being in some far-flung part of the globe with shaky mobile coverage: 'Please leave a message after your moan.'

Dirk, to give him his due, *was* in the country when my GP advised at just shy of eight weeks that an immediate hospital trip was wise 'in case you're losing your baby'. In case I'm losing my baby? Howl!

Dirk was there to help me through the mire of being boomeranged back and forth between A&E or the EPU with a firm 'Look, can someone just see us? Now?' He was there to hold my hand in the waiting room amidst pregnant women with noisy, kicking, breathing, *alive* children at their ankles. And he was there to grimace manfully when I finally went in for my first taster of the pregnant woman's undignified lot at the hands of the medical profession. Cold, begloved, invading hands. An internal probe. Octave-jumping, knee-jerk response from yours truly. Literally.

And while I coughed and tried to coax my voice back into a comfortable register, all of a sudden there it was. A tiny but unmistakable pinprick of life. Flash, flash, flashing on the screen. It was a minuscule speck. But it was alive!

'Aren't you glad you were in the country now?' I squeaked.

I shuffled off the bed and the sonographer discreetly pulled a curtain across while I stepped back into my underwear. It was kind of her to pretend she hadn't just seen me in all my glory, both inside and out.

I staggered off out of the consulting room. I felt like one of those traditional wooden toy animals you used to get, that would go all floppy when you pressed the base it stood on. I *had* been standing tall on my neat little podium, pleased as punch with what life had thrown my way. And then suddenly, someone had rammed their thumbs up inside my plinth and my legs had collapsed without warning. After a bit of light toying around, the thumbs had eventually been withdrawn. My limbs had sprung obediently back into place. But I was still, to be honest, feeling a bit wobbly.

All this I had kept hidden from my mum. Why? At the time when I needed her most, I'd drawn a veil across our affairs.

Later on, I'd tell her of my pregnancies almost immediately. But that first time, Dirk and I had implicitly agreed to keep a lid on it. Wanting to pull a surprise out of the bag? Not wishing to tempt fate? Wanting to have something secret just for us for a bit?

It reminded me of butterfly-catching as a kid. We had an enormous Buddleia bush at the front of our house that attracted butterflies like boys to a steam train. I was the proud possessor of a long-handled blue nylon net and with it I'd go out on the hunt for Peacocks, Red Admirals and Cabbage Whites. On a good day, I'd capture one or two and incarcerate them in a customised jam jar made homely with a snapped-off leaf and some accommodating air vents. I'd press my nose to the glass of my hostages' temporary home and try to fight off the creeping feeling that it was a bit wrong. I must have eventually let them free before bedtime as I can't recall ever having to dispose of a butterfly corpse.

I *do* however remember once imprisoning a clutch of caterpillars, keen to watch the butterfly life cycle unfold beneath my very eyes. I'd stuffed in some lettuce, furnished the lid with plenty of air holes and stashed the jar expectantly under my bed. To no avail. When I awoke in the morning it was with horror that I discovered my ventilation holes had been too big. The creepies had crawled out overnight. I was both gutted and afflicted by the raving itches. I swear I didn't sleep for weeks. The butterfly population had wreaked its revenge.

It's the end of the evening. I yawn. Captive butterflies in jam jars seem distant. If we hang around much longer Santa and his airborne friends will soon be nigh.

It's been a good night. Full of good cheer and expectation. I wonder how different next Christmas will be. Very, I think. In the meantime, I consider if it would be too bad form to play my pregnancy card. I yawn again and think, well why not?

'By the way,' I say, scraping back my chair. 'Did I mention? All I want for Christmas is my two pans scrubbed. Goodnight!' And on that note I make a not very decorous run for it.

Chapter 2

Christmas, being Christmas, only lasted one day, and now here we are swinging into 2002. Usually, New Years are about new hope, new diets and new headaches, courtesy of the wrath of grapes. But as we turn into this one, my head is clear of fuzz, like a puffed-off dandelion clock. I laugh in the face of my usual mind-over-platter January resolutions. And I am full, quite literally, of the hope of new life.

My diary, by comparison, looks ominously light. The Big Event is still miles off of course. D-Day is not till the summer. Pregnancy, I now know, ekes out over forty *very* long weeks. I know this because I am now in the club. I know that you do not, sheesh, count pregnancy in months. Who *does* that anyway?

So the months – sorry, the weeks – ahead look fairly blank. This is not because I have no friends, let me assure you. Anyway, nobody ever does anything in January, do they? And even if they are, after negotiating my first pregnant Christmas, I'm feeling a bit thick and tired to be honest. Well, that's my excuse and I'm sticking to it.

And besides, at the moment, everything else that is not to do with my pregnancy has dropped off my radar. News, politics, music and gossip all seem to have faded into also-ran insignificance. Who gives a monkey's about all of that when there's something far more important to focus on?

I

a m

p r e

gnant. Wh

ich is really qu

ite exciting. Doesn

't the world agree? Not

that the world knows yet. Not much of it.

My reference points are now, when is the next scan? When is it safe to tell everyone else? When can I start shopping?

Except in reality my life isn't a series of blank squares you can skip through until the interesting bits come along. The humdrum stops for no one. I still need to drag myself through the short term. To eat, drink, sleep and clock in and out of work. (And when the clock gets hungry I go back four seconds.)

Work. I work at BA under the marketing department umbrella.

Sitting under that umbrella means I have occasionally to

shelter from the odd squally jargon spell. Don't think I find these a problem; there is no such thing as a problem, just a range of fresh challenges. Saying that, I do find it useful having a brolly to hand at all times. I need it as protection against the continual drizzle of irritating phrases like 'paradigm shift', 'cash cows', 'low-hanging fruit' and 'let's touch bases offline'. Oh, and of course to weather all the brain storms.

Fortunately, I steer well clear of strategising and anything too technically demanding or borderline nerdy. My corner of the department, production, works on the words and pictures and colour mix on the website, interactive TV and WAP phones. Oh, and we do our bit on the coffee-vending machine, which gets a serious hammering after a team-building night out. When the digital display reads 'Out of Order' you know the team is also at risk of serious malfunction if they don't score a decent caffeine fix soon.

The production team seems remarkably free of anyone with kids of their own. We are all fairly young, we make frequent use of our knock-down flight concessions and our ability to travel at the drop of a hat, and I'd be willing to wager none of us at this point has even heard of Gina Ford.

But the morning after I found out that I was pregnant, that *I* was now different, all that, for the time being, had to be kept secret. Nobody could know. It was still too early. This in spite of the fact that my demeanour must surely have been a little unusual given that my whole world had turned upside down overnight.

Whilst my body was busy welcoming in its new forty-week guest with a well-stocked minibar, a fluffy dressing gown and a Gideon Bible in the drawer, my head felt as though it was whirling round like the water draining down the plughole in the en-suite next door.

I'd driven into work head spinning, grinning to myself in delight and desperately trying to keep my feet on the ground. It was important to pretend that nothing had changed. I must make sure I act normally at all times. I inched along the Euston Road and wondered how I'd do it. And as I drove on through Hammersmith and down the Great West Road past Chiswick I put together a little checklist on how to get through the day without spilling the beans. It went something like this:

Follow the I'm Not Pregnant, No Really I'm Not Code

- Enjoy the office and respect the right of hot desks to remain unlittered with crumbs just because you're eating for two now
- Guard against all risk of fiery blushes should anyone mention projects due for delivery in the next forty or so weeks
- Close all toilet doors. Do not, whatever you do, leave with your skirt tucked into your tights
- Keep your gushes about the beauty of new life under close control
- Keep to well-trodden paths and avoid the smokers' corner
- Use stairs and lifts to avoid eaters of falafel, haggis or smelly egg sandwiches which are sure to make you sick as a dog
- Leave your aching breasts alone – someone's bound to notice
- Take your pregnancy mag home
- Help to keep all discussion free of references to fluffy birds or kittens – it's anyone's guess how your treacherous hormones will respond
- Protect your computer screen from idle snoopers. Do not, whatever you do, let them see you surfing baby-clothes sites
- Take special care walking downstairs – they say your balance will be affected

- Make no unnecessary noise, i.e. keep your trap shut before you blurt it out and give the game away

As I rolled into the underground car park that November morning, I allowed myself a smug smile. That just about covers all bases. I should be fine. No one will know a thing. I grabbed my bag, locked the car and headed for the stairs up the ground level.

'All right, Charlotte. How's it going?' said a voice over my left shoulder.

'Oh, all right, Charlie? Fine, thanks,' I replied with false nonchalance. This cover-up operation is going to be a breeze.

'A bit in the clouds today are we?' he went on.

'No. Er. Why?' I asked offhand, stooping to retrieve the ID card that had clattered perfidiously to the floor.

'It's just that you've got your top on inside out. Look. I can see your label.'

'Sheesh. Easy mistake to make,' I said, not adding 'when your head's inside out too'.

Damn. Two minutes down and I'd already blown my cover.

In those early weeks of confirmed pregnancy, I'd felt ... well, confused, frankly. According to my calculations I was now four weeks pregnant. But according to the doctor I was six weeks. How would he know? He wasn't there!

When I went to the GP to declare my pregnancy I confess I was expecting a little more than I actually got. A small fanfare, a pat on the back, a big fat tick in the box from the guy with the hallmarks of an important person – the medical qualifications, an impressive-looking shiny thing round his neck, his surname printed grandly on a plaque – to confirm that, yes, I was indeed pregnant. In fact, first of all, I got little more than an enquiring silence.

23

'How can I help you today, Mrs Moerman?'

'Well, I think I'm pregnant.'

'?'

'Erm, I thought, I mean I've read, well, actually, I've probably seen on the TV that you need to, erm, go along to your GP?'

'Well, you've come to the right place, here I am. But I just need to establish ... am I to congratulate or commiserate?'

'Oh blimey, yes. I suppose you do, don't you? Well, yes, this is very much a wanted pregnancy, thanks.'

'Good, good. Well, we'll just take down a few dates then and check your blood pressure and then you should get a booking-in appointment letter from the hospital for about six weeks' time, all being well.'

No fanfare. No back pats. Not even a measly urine test. I'd been hoping for a physical check to prove I wasn't just making it all up. How impending motherhood has changed me. I actually *wanted* the doc to ask me to step into the cubicle, remove my lower garments and make myself comfortable on the couch. As if.

But he didn't and I didn't. We just had our cosy little chat while I filled in some forms, I had the inflatable cuff velcroed round my upper arm and then I was dismissed.

I went out empty-handed, at best a little crestfallen. OK, maybe I was expecting too much – a sealed-with-wax crested certificate, a herald of trumpets – but at the very least I'd kind of hoped for a dry-cleaning-type chitty to take in and redeem at the hospital in due course. That'd be an idea eh?

Your GP:	An NHS one – won't take you to the cleaners
Address:	Grotty but serviceable surgery
No. of pieces:	One, soon to be two. Or could be three, who knows?
Item:	Mum-to-be. Plus baby/babies (see above)

Cash:	Nothing to pay today. 'Tis but a matter of time ...
Date:	November 2001. For collection ... August some time?
Ref:	DS/DD 2 B

Alas there were none of these. Not even a rudimentary check and a verbal confirmation that I was indeed expecting. I'd just have to wait a little while longer, it seemed, for the verification I craved. Though not a full six weeks as it turned out.

The spotting which had plagued me soon receded and I was grateful to no longer have to describe the size of the staining in my pants to people I'd only just had the pleasure of meeting. 'Five pence, fifty pence or a twenty-pound note, in which case you're really in trouble.'

I focused instead on coming blissfully to terms with my change in status. Dirk slotted ostensibly straight back into his routine, gadding about all over the globe. I too was entering hitherto unexplored domains, treading new routes through local places I mistakenly thought I knew. I went to the newsagent and discovered a rack of pregnancy mags, which I'd swear were never there before. I went along with my demanding new pregnancy bladder into more public toilets than I knew existed, or ever wanted to know existed. And I became acquainted with a whole new aisle in the supermarket that had never before tickled my fancy. Who drinks fruit teas other than pregnant or breastfeeding women, I wonder? With a cupboard still stashed full of the stuff I'm still trying to find that one out, actually.

Aside from my blind date with the Twinings aisle, I stumbled into an obsessive new fascination with identifying those around me who were, or seemed to be, pregnant. Just as when I'd broken my ankle and suddenly noticed all manner of people struggling around London Transport on crutches like myself, freakily, now that I was expecting, it seemed that half the population had buns in the oven. Well, not half, obviously, or it'd mean that every single female from cradle to the coffin queue was up the duff, but you know what I mean.

I, of course, wasn't showing at this stage. But I couldn't help but think that it was obvious to all that, like the accents in the Abba songs or old ladies' blue-rinse hairdos, something wasn't quite right with me. This was before the days of 'Baby on Board' badges on coats, so Tube seat squatters had to guess if you looked pregnant and peaky, or just fat and hungover.

Compared with some I was relatively blessed as I escaped the curse of morning sickness. Neither did I go off certain foods or suffer slow torture by the ancient method of heartburn. Instead I was afflicted by the raciest dreams you could contemplate (some might see this as a positive boon). I was, naturally, quick to respond to Mother Nature's ploy to fatten up her newly expectant mum, and I was extraordinarily, unbelievably tired.

This was a special kind of tiredness reserved for early pregnancy, unlike anything I'd ever felt before. At this stage I was a mere novice in the field of different types of tiredness, mind. Later on, there'd be the physical tiredness of being unable to sleep properly with That Bump to negotiate at night, the emotional tiredness of agonising if the unborn baby was OK, and the mental tiredness of batting off this person and that each with an opinion on every aspect of your pregnancy, your lifestyle ('You're eating *tomatoes!*') and your choice of potential names and/or your decision not to share your list of potential names. It would be exhausting. And then the baby would arrive. And then another. And then another. By the end of three lots of pregnancies, births and baby years, not to mention managing the ensuing rugby scrum, I would eventually mature into an Inuit tribeswoman with 300 ways to describe being knackered.

Inspecting my wan face in the mirror, I wondered how the celebrities did it. The recently delivered Davina McCall always seemed to me to be almost indecently perky and very much awake. When the newly expectant Liz Hurley peeked out from behind her Gucci sunglasses she looked, as far as I could tell, not a bit hollow-eyed or drawn. And the pregnant Jordan? Well she was a law unto her own, but one thing's for sure, for her looking knackered was always going to be off limits.

But anyway who cared about them? They weren't 'real'. Not like you or me. I'd never risen to the bait of comparing myself to these glamour women before I conceived so why should it be any different now that we had a mutual pregnancy thing in common?

Instead I consoled myself with images of more down-to-earth mums of our time who restored faith in the fact that, yes, it was OK to look knackered. And in some cases very knackered. Thanks, Cherie, you didn't half give me a lift sometimes.

Chapter 3

We're a few weeks into 2002. The room feels hot and stuffy in spite of it being January. In the seat next to me Dirk is fidgeting. For someone who's used to sitting still for hours at a time on a plane, he seems remarkably twitchy. Perhaps he's waiting for someone in a uniform to come along and offer him a drink and then he'll calm down. But today the drinks are on, or in, me.

It's 11.37. Our appointment was at 11 a.m. So was the appointment for the handful of other expectant mums sitting uncomfortably in the aptly named waiting room. Except those whose appointments were at 10.30.

Some are sitting hand-in-hand with a partner or husband, occasionally sharing a hushed comment or time-check grumble. One has her own mother with her, and a handful of noisy children at her feet. To my right in the corner is a Muslim couple sitting still and dignified, her face partly hidden by a pale mauve veil. To my left is a woman clearly nipping in between meetings, dressed in a suit, sitting alone and tapping notes on a handheld PDA. What is she writing? I muse to myself to pass the time – 'RSVP – no can do – launch party drinks Tuesday week'? 'Conference, Athens, June'? 'www.Mothercare.com'?

We're a motley bunch from a variety of ages, stages and walks of life. But we've all got a few things in common. First and foremost, we're all here for our twelve-week booking-in scan. We've all obediently filled in the NHS forms and, on pain of a verbal lashing, returned the pencils to the receptionist. We've all sat flicking through the tattered magazines, most of which date from the last decade. And we've all gazed listlessly around the room at the no mobile phones sign, the – ugh – scan picture of twins (!) and the TV playing silently to itself in the corner above our heads. And last but not least, and perhaps most pressingly of all, we're all bursting for the loo.

Our appointment cards had instructed us to arrive having drunk a good slug of water. This is ostensibly so that your bladder is full and pushes the baby into a better viewing position. That, however, is a load of codswallop. The real reason for asking you to knock back a couple of pints of Evian is to provide some light relief for the sourpusses who sit at Reception whose days would otherwise be an unbroken litany of 'Yes, we're running a little late. You're next/twelfth/thirty-third on the list. No, you can't go to the toilet yet.'

Cut forward a few years and I'm the one with a couple of noisy kids at my feet. I've not OD'd on the water this time. I'm a seasoned professional. I am a goddess of calm. I am Bjorn Borg, cool as ice before a match-point serve. I am as relaxed as Frankie on his way to Hollywood. I am cool as the proverbial cucumber. I *can* hold my bladder this time and I *will not* get ruffled.

Until one of my sons knocks a plastic cup of water over the floor and the other starts shooting an imaginary gun at the assembled silent crowd. A toy is trodden on. A menacing shriek is let loose. Quickly followed by another, which soon morphs into a low, plaintive moan, a wretched backing-track to our drawn-out wait.

The receptionist gives me the evils over her spectacles. A clearly first-time mum looks on, alarmed.

I hush the boys, take a limp sip at my warm bottle of water and shift uncomfortably on my no longer cool and goddess-like buttocks.

'Are we nearly there?' whispers Dirk in my ear.

All this painful sitting about, legs crossed, willing for someone to call out my mispronounced name is of course nothing but a luxury.

In Mum's time, there weren't any scans to determine whether you really were expecting one, two or a fistful of babies and certainly no magic ways of seeing inside the womb to check if baby was healthy, two-headed or likely to inherit its father's nose.

I think back to Mum, pregnant with her first child, as good as alone in Canada. My parents had married and transferred their lives there, a long way from British friends and family back home. What must it have been like for her?

It was 1970. Unrest was all around. Europe had witnessed the Sorbonne marches and the Baader-Meinhof gang. Now the Northern American young were rioting over Vietnam, and protesting students in Chicago Kent State University were shot by federal troops. The innocence of flower power was behind. For my newly pregnant mum, it was very much a time for growing up.

Skip forward to the 1980s. Braintree, Essex. Mum, now a senior radiographer with a crisp white coat, Dr Scholl's footwear and a formidable lead jacket for when the going got tough, decided to extend her repertoire. When the opportunity arose to retrain in the new, cutting-edge Ultrasound technology, she jumped in with both cork-soled, leather-buckled, comfortably clad feet.

With the aid of this shrewd new technology, Mum was one of the first to embark on a new mission, to explore the strange new world of Essex Woman's Tum. To seek out the new life within and the promise of new civilisation. Boldly going where no woman had gone before, she negotiated the unchartered territory of a thousand pregnant bellies with the aid of a simple brick-like device. It was as sleek as an early mobile phone, but it did the job. And with it, she peered into swollen wombs aplenty, looking for pointy Vulcan ears, ridged Klingon foreheads and worse.

Tellingly, Mum always said that on learning how many things could go wrong in unborn babies, she was glad she'd stopped at two. I took this to mean she didn't consider me as a baby that had 'gone wrong', though I often wonder if I continued to live up to expectations as her child and now as an adult.

I take another slurp in spite of myself. Wouldn't do to get in, find I hadn't drunk quite enough and be made to do the walk of shame back to the waiting room with a red face and a fresh flagon of water in my fist.

'Do you really need to keep drinking? You've had quite a lot,' frowns Dirk.

'They said two litres. I think. Anyway, better safe than sorry,' I hiss defensively back.

'Merm ...? More ... man? Eugh ... Charlotte?'

'Yup. That's me!'

Gathering together my handbag, my crumpled *Metro* and a clutch of spent Evian bottles, I spring up all of a panic, anxious not to miss my turn. Dirk, sucking in his teeth at either a) the Anna Friel/Darren Day spread in the 1994 issue of *Hello!* or b) the amount of time we've been kept hanging on (you be the judge) trails in noiselessly behind me.

I am lying on the bed. The strip light is buzzing. There's a straggled end of tinsel still sellotaped to a corner of the ceiling. Dirk smiles his encouragement.

'Right Mrs M— can I call you Charlotte?' says the sonographer, 'let's have a little look at this baby shall we?'

She picks up a washing-up-type bottle and shakes it vigorously up and down. I feel like a plate of chips about to get doused in ketchup.

'Sorry, there's a heater for the gel in the other room, but you might just find this one a little ...'

COLD! I don't hear the end of her sentence as the chilly gloop hits my hitherto winter-warmed belly. My taut bladder squeals in dismay. So do I when the sonographer says 'Oh my, that *is* a full bladder isn't it? I'll need you to pop out to the loo and empty it just *a little*.'

I'm beginning to dislike this woman and her littles.

Dirk shuffles deeper into the room remaining tactfully silent. He may have growled at the receptionists but he knows better than to utter another word at this point. There's a hint of a smile playing treacherously on his lips. He doesn't need to say anything, though. I hate it when he's right.

I swing my legs off the bed, slip out and find a nearby toilet. Never has a grotty hospital loo seemed more welcoming. Although, of course, at this point in time I'm unable to fully enjoy the benefits. 'Just *a little*,' I remind myself before I'm tempted to unleash Niagara. A stack of sample bottles sits tauntingly at eye level. It's like a maths problem at school: 'If a woman has capacity to fill thirty-three urine jars but may only fill five of them, how many jars' worth of urine will still be squeezed into her bursting bladder?'

I climb back onto the bed. I pull down my now gel-soggy maternity trousers. The roller-ball joystick is reapplied. I'm feverishly excited. The sonographer cranes towards the screen. White shapes flicker across the screen. It's virtually silent and I'm in utter awe.

'There it is. That's your baby. Now I'm just going to take a few measurements.'

I nod my interview-technique encouraging nod, except, of course, I'm lying down unclothed rather than sitting perkily upright in my interview suit. We'd seen the beating pinprick before Christmas. Though it had been amazing it was, let's be honest, just a dot. Now, only a few weeks later, it is indisputably a baby. There's the heartbeat. There's the head. And there's the tail. Tail? It looks like I'm giving birth to a mythical creature of the deep, part-human, part-shrimp.

Later on, when we attend the scans for our second and then third children, I'm seriously underwhelmed at this point. Once you've seen the twenty-weeker with what looks like a 'proper' baby, the twelve-week job in subsequent iterations is ... well ... a bit like a Hollywood sequel: OK, still amazing, but not as good as the original. But, pah, forget what Dirk and I think, what do our wide-eyed little henchmen make of their first eyeful of *Prawn Child: the Movie*? What were they were expecting – full Technicolor digital cinema with surround-sound? A jolly Mr Tumble signing out something special which is either very friendly and helpful, or deeply insulting depending on your viewpoint? A waving baby sibling? But no, there's none of that. No colour, no music, nothing obviously baby-like other than that ghostly football that they claim is the head. Mindful of my feelings after I've bigged the visit up, they don't directly say it's been pants. Instead, they simply pull for the door mewling 'Is it finished now?' and 'Can we go? I need the toilet!'

Back through the mists of time, and the original sonographer is saying 'The measurements all look normal.'

(Normal for a child-crustacean that is.) 'But I've seen a little something in the brain that'll need a follow-up appointment.'

I know instantly that this is not a little something but a huge and significant something. I know I must be brave. My eyes prick, I glaze over and I let Dirk pick up the slack, talking about what this might mean and what happens next while I hover in the background like a moth at a night light.

I feel a chill across my naked belly. The high-tech machinery buzzes darkly. I take the proffered roll of blue paper, mop a bit of clear liquid off my skin and restore my trousers to waist-height. I hear the sonographer saying 'It's probably nothing, these things usually disappear, but we do have to check. Make an appointment for ten days and we'll see if the shadow's still there then.' She packs us off with an explanatory piece of paper. 'No need to worry for now.'

No need to worry. Who's she trying to kid? My stomach is in knots, I have a cold sweat on and I am convinced that from this very moment in time I will worry my socks off every waking hour and then some.

This, I now know, is parenthood for you.

Back to the future and I've graduated. I am a parent of three. I now have a degree in worrying.

BSc (Hons) Parental Anxiety. Course Code: ROFL NOT
You need: 360 points and nerves of steel
Level: Undergraduate
Description:
If you're awarded a BSc (Hons) in Parental Anxiety you'll understand the ideas, theories, methods and debates in parental angst. You'll be able to analyse and evaluate the concepts and theories behind why we willingly enter into

this thing called parenthood, which invariably reduces us to a bundle of nerves. And you'll be able to assess different kinds of bloody worrying episodes including quantitative and qualitative examples of being worried sick.

Studying Parental Anxiety can help you find answers to questions like these:

- Why can't I remember what it was like not to have children to worry about?
- What impact does my eternally frazzled disposition have on my children?
- How did I become who I am – and who was I in the first place anyway?
- How do I know if I'm doing it right?

Practical assignments include:

- Pregnancy scans ending in tears (at least 2)
- Nocturnal calls to NHS Direct, followed by madcap hospital dashes with sheet-white child in arms (3)
- Disciplinary measures undertaken ending in tears (children in tears – 37, mother in tears – 164)
- Stomach-churning lurches at discovery of child's awkwardness in the social morass of the playground (quite a few), and at own awkwardness (quite a few too)
- Sleepless nights over amount of time child is spending in front of telly, up to their ears in chocolate, duvet-surfing down the stairs etc (lots)
- Comedy double takes at cash point after spending not a little on nappies, limited edition Frubes and lorry-

loads of *essential* cheap-sellotaped-on-gimmick comics
(more than I care to mention)

Actually, you know that bit about me saying I've graduated.
Well, just ignore that bit. Technically speaking, I'm not quite
ready to pose for the photo in a gown, a mortarboard and a
particularly bad hairdo yet.

I've been great at immersing myself in the practical side of
things. But I'm buggered if I understand it.

Ten, long days later, and we're back. Today we're being seen by
a senior sonographer with an attentive bedside manner and a
name I have no hope of being able to pronounce. I feel we
instantly have a bond.

He leads us into the consulting room. I lie down, prepared
this time for a cold shock. I'm pleasantly surprised, however,
when a warm goo hits the decks. It reminds me of the inviting
tepid ooze of mud pies. I remark to myself how we've gone up in
the world, scoring both the charming consultant and the room
with the gel-warming gadget. Maybe things are looking up?

He swivels round the monitor so I get a ringside view without
having to crane my neck like a contortionist. It's a little like
those Magic Eye 3D pictures with all those crazily coloured dots
that revealed a hidden image to those with the right kind of
squint. I narrow my eyes and scrutinise the screen. If I look hard
enough perhaps it might make sense.

'Your baby appears to be doing brilliantly,' says the
consultant. He can obviously do this parallel viewing thing
then. I'm still struggling. So the baby's doing brilliantly. At
what? Wallowing gracefully in the warm waters like a
therapeutic tourist, executing a nifty length or two of fused-leg
foetus butterfly, rubbing its tummy and patting its head whilst

making a cup of tea? I don't know and I don't care about any of this. I just want to find out if there's still a shadow in the left ventricle of its brain.

'What about the shadow?'

'Well, I've had a good look and you'll be pleased to hear I can't see anything,' he says. 'Of course, nothing's one hundred per cent certain until the fat lady sings. But from what I can see today, this baby of yours is progressing absolutely normally. For now at least, this little one's doing just fine.'

I'm pleased, of course, with this verdict. And I would like to sing like a fat and enormously relieved lady. But I can't shake off the niggling doubt that seems to have settled on me like the layer of dust on the mags in the waiting room.

· · ·

An Invitation!

What:	Please join Claudia, Andrew and Chloe Charlotte for a Baby Viewing Party!
When:	Saturday 2 March 2002 at 2 p.m., if we're out of our PJs by then!
Bring:	Yourselves and your sympathetic faces. With sore bits like mine, I need all the sympathy I can get!
Directions:	Drive to the usual address. Ring on the door. Come in. Might be a bit messy. Hormonal late-pregnancy nesting blitz has fizzled.
RSVP:	Claudia (aka Mummy!), preferably by email. Phone conversations being currently limited to the likes of 'Me Knackered, you Jane.'

Come Join the Fun!

Tuesday morning, just after the Fat Lady scan. Today I am glowing like the Ready Brek kid. Thin wintery sunshine filters through the permanently sealed windows. The open-plan office is a hive of activity. It's reminiscent of a familiar scene of industry which hung on the wall above our phone at home when I was a kid.

There are matchstick men on phones, on laptops, on their way to or from the loo. There are matchstick men in glass-walled meeting rooms, brainstorming on flip charts, conference calling in huddles or thoughtfully chewing at Bic biros. There are men with 'Have you seen Del's joke in your inbox?' grins, men tinkering gleefully with their latest mobile gadget, and men with hair at various stages of thinning.

Admittedly, these particular matchstick men are a little different from the folk of Salford in the first half of the twentieth century. They're enjoying the benefits of central heating, mixed company and a free coffee-vending machine for starters. And they're neither accompanied by matchstick cats or dogs, nor any miscellaneous kids hanging round the periphery in clogs either. (Unless you count the burgeoning half Dutch one in my tummy that is.)

Still, it's a comforting idea and I'm (match) sticking to it.

I'm happy because my baby is OK. I can at last share the news with my friends and colleagues. And I can slough off the despondency that has of late beset me. I always thought the baby blues were supposed to come post-natally but I've already had a fortnight's worth of bad heir days.

Later on, I would immerse myself amongst matchstick women and matchstick kids at toddler drop-in groups. They'd be crawling, sitting and hammering plastic infant activity toys (batteries long expired) on every available surface. There would be a famine of men unless you counted Bob the Builder in the toy bucket. And he wasn't all there, having lost an arm somewhere out on active service.

No wonder there's a dearth of dads, though. I have to say it would worry me if I was a bloke considering entering this room; women gossiping at full tilt, children running amok, grinding biscuits into the carpet and invariably *at least* one ponging. And what would you do in the event of a fire when, in thick smoke and panicking, all the women and children would hotfoot out the room first and you'd be abandoned with the one-armed bandit trying to fend off the flames.

'Can we quench it?' 'No we can't.' Not with only two useful fanning arms, one highly meltable plastic one, and another which has long since gone AWOL. (I always reckoned those break-dancing moves in the vid for 'Mambo No. 5' were a bit too ambitious for you, Bob.)

I take a sip of my lukewarm tea. It's pretty horrible to be honest, but it's free and we all drink it, because, well, you just do don't you? It's reminiscent of my career path, come to think of it. I did what I had to at school, went to university and then hopped into white-collar work because ... because what? It was what everyone did? It was expected of me? It was a chance to belong, to be told I was doing OK.

And so here I am with my white-ridged, disposable cup of char. I'm at ease. My dark mood has lifted. And I no longer need to hide a stonking great secret from my friends and colleagues. Which of my colleagues to tell first? And how?

I swing my chair back round to face the monitor. My fingers make contact with the keys and I try to wrench my mind back on to the job in hand for now. Now where's my to do list? Let's see:

i)   Review PIR questionnaires on the new workflow
ii) Proofread revised ICG standards copy
iii) Try out a couple of PFEs (Pelvic Floor Exercises)

Pelvic Floor Exercises, I'm told, are the way forward. Or, more precisely, the way to avoid everything going downward.

I'd always been more of an artsy kind of girl rather than swaying towards the sciences or ... shudder ... mathematical pursuits. I remember in Biology drawing the painstaking anatomy of a Daffodil, gagging through a rat dissection and giggling with the rest when it came to Sex Ed. I don't however recall GCSE Biology making reference to Pelvic Floor Muscles. Correct me if I'm wrong, but I don't think the humble Daff had them. Though the rat may have done, I wasn't getting close enough to find out. And none of us, let's face it, were focusing on the Pelvic Floor area when it came to the human reproduction diagrams.

So this apparently quite important Pelvic Floor stuff is, like the herbal teas, another new concept to explore and abhor. I squeeze in and up and feel my face must express the look of a freshly stung Joyce Grenfell trying to keep it all together in front of a roomful of St Trinian's gels.

I'm supposed to fit these into my daily routine and do them without anyone noticing. I've resolved to try doing them whenever I answer the phone, stop at traffic lights or spot a magpie. The phone rings. I pick it up and launch into conversation.

Rats! I think to myself as I chatter distractedly with my colleague. Almost forgot. I pull up my right buttock half-heartedly but I know I'm not doing it right. Still, at least I've got more lower-torso muscle mobility than the long-deceased rodent.

• • •

Instructions Not Included

While I'm determinedly sucking everything in so that I can sneeze without mishap in the years ahead, Dirk's letting it all hang out on a business-class seat to Hong Kong.

He's less concerned about sneezing fluids out than absorbing up the new. He's like that. A sponge. He once picked up some sort of malarial bug from his far-flung travels that left him faint and nauseous for weeks. He's soaked up more variants of Heineken's global portfolio of beers than you can shake a stick at. And he's learned to say 'please' and 'thank you' and 'Where's the taxi rank?' in more languages than you care to imagine.

The term Frequent Flier was invented for him. He has more stamps in his passport than a Stanley Gibbons catalogue. He's probably been to more countries than a good many pilots. And he's an Air Miles mile-o-naire. I've been about a lot too, though business travel has waned for me of late. Still, it would be no good for my PFEs up there (traffic lights in the clouds, anyone?), so it's probably just as well, really.

Wouldn't it be nice to be poured into one of those plaster-of-Paris craft kits I used to love? I did Peter Rabbit once and I'm sure I gave Mrs Tiggy-Winkle a go, though the spikes must have been a bit of a challenge. You'd take the bag of plaster, mix with water and stir, and then you'd pour the gloop into the mould of your choice. You'd leave it to set, then peel off the mould, sand a bit for perfection and paint. Then ... ta da ... you'd have a perfect little plaster model to sit and gather dust on your bedroom shelf.

I'd like to feel that we'll get mixed up with a confident stir and then poured together into the happy family mould. What you'd get at the end is a picture-perfect figurine that depicts a three-way hug between newborn and adoring parents. There'd be no chips, or sticking-out bits where the plaster seeped through the mould, and the heady-smelling paint would all be perfectly applied.

Sounds great. But somehow it never quite turns out like the example on the box.

I frown determinedly at the screen and cross one ankle over the other. A tangled twine of network cables emerges from a customised hole in the carpet tiles at my feet. It reminds me of Rapunzel's hair, a thick rope offering me the chance of – what – escape? Or just beckoning me to come back down to earth.

My line manager saunters past, reminding me of the task in hand. Forget airy-fairy thoughts of grasping a rope ladder made of hair, now's the time to seize the opportunity to break the news of my delicate state to my boss.

The thing is, I'm quite enjoying this being in limbo. I know things are, supposedly, A-OK now with the baby. And I'm back on an even keel emotionally. Things seem back to normal. But as soon as I share my news, I can't then just act normally any more. Because everything will have changed. And if everything has changed, will I still belong, or will I already effectively be making my way out the door?

Oh, stuff it. Time to bite the bullet.

'Erm, Caryn ... there's something I need to talk to you about. Can we grab five minutes?'

'Sure. I'm pretty chocka, but have a look in my diary and send me an invite. I think I've got some space tomorrow first thing.'

'Well, I'd quite like to see you soon. It'll only take five minutes, promise.'

Caryn was always in a rush. Her slight wiry frame bore testament to the fact that she rarely stood still. I couldn't imagine her slender frame pregnant whereas I'd always known that my body would happily adapt to maternity in a full-on big, blousy way. If she's the angular speed-cloud inducing Mr Rush,

I'm Mr Greedy's rotund pink blob. And that's before I'm even in my second trimester.

'Grab me at the end of the day, then,' she gabbles over her shoulder as she dashes off to another meeting. 'I'm back-to-back till sixish, but I can fit you in after then.' And she's off on her whirlwind of meetings, phone calls and cigarette breaks.

I sit back down at my temporary desk relieved I've now got a timeline on breaking the news. It's a hot-desking office, though like children in the classroom we often gravitate back to the same place out of habit. I wonder how much longer I'll be haring across London each morning in order to arrive in time to cadge my favourite place.

Hmm, I know, let's play spot the difference. Yes let's!

Here's how it goes. There's a page bursting with cheerful primaries and jolly bubble writing. There are two large, similar-looking pictures printed side by side.

On the first picture, there's a woman in crisp suit, smiling and holding a laptop bag, a mobile phone and a loadsa money wad of notes. In the second picture is a woman in tired jeans, she's grimacing and holding a baby. There's a toddler clinging to her ankles and a third child sneaking off with her (practically empty) purse.

You have to:

1) Look closely at the two pictures. How many differences can you spot in picture 2?
2) Stick some stickers over the gaps in picture 2 and see if you can fudge it to seem more like picture 1. (No idea why, but stickers always seem to help.)
3) Look closely again at picture 1. How many things do you think you simply can't fudge back with stickers?

4) Which picture do you prefer?

5) Give yourself a sticker!

Hmm, bit tricky this one. Let's take a closer look. Oh, no I've got it, they're two utterly and completely different people! No similarities at all. Nyet, nada, nothing! (Do I still get the sticker at the end?)

But hang on a minute, not so fast wise guy. Let's look again. I feel a list coming on ...

1.i) In that first picture, our woman is a form-filler-inner – forms for booking meeting rooms, applications for leave, 360-degree reviews, staff travel requests, expense claims, project specifications, best-practice checklists, post-implementation reviews ... zzzz ... orders for lunch anyone?

1.ii) In the second picture, our doughty lass is, what's this, *still* filling in forms for school dinners, school uniform and subsidised cycling helmets. She's got Rainbow Day sponsorship forms, forms for the Children's Flower Society annual Daffodil-growing competition, and she spends not inconsiderable time finding a slot on the forms for the up-and-coming parents' evening. When she will be going over the forms that the teacher's been filling in on the subject of her child for OFSTED. Forms, it seems are the norm.

2.i) Picture 1 again. Here our woman, a Project Manager through and through, spends her time sniffing out effective short cuts to help her deliver on target, in time, gun smoking. She reckons she's a pretty ace multi-tasker.

2.ii) Picture 2. Surprise! This woman eats short cuts for breakfast. She swears allegiance to Delia, Queen of all Store Cupboard Ingredients. She wears only non-iron clothes or very crinkled cotton ones. And she fabricates pledges on the kids' sponsored Let's Sting Mummy Again forms (who ever goes around and asks *real* people anyway?). She *thought* she was a multi-tasker. And then she became a mum.

3.i) This woman smartly uses the resources available to keep herself and her kit prepped and ready for duty. She has PDA, mobile and laptop chargers handy at all times. Strong coffees on tap, and after-work beers frequently advisable.

3.ii) This woman desperately uses the resources available frantically to try keeping herself above water. She keeps carbs, Ribena and Cheese Strings in the cupboards at all times. Stiff drinks before bedtime (sometimes quite a long time before bedtime) essential.

4.i) This woman keeps track of her expenses and stays on top of her budget.

4ii) This woman keeps abreast of ELC bargains and blanks out her expenditure on cakes and cappuccinos in Starbucks.

5.i) This woman sings to herself late at night when the office is nearly empty. She gets up and down to activate the movement-sensitive lights. She's tempted to get up and dance occasionally too. She doesn't. She listens to Crapital in the car on the long commute home in the dark, reheats a meal, and collapses into bed.

5.ii) This woman sing sing sings more than she ever thought humanly possible when she used to listen to Travis crooning the most played hit of summer 2001 in the car on her late commutes home to an often empty house. Only she doesn't sing the stuff of Fran Healy these days (unless he's ever done a remake of 'Twinkle Twinkle' that I missed?). Her kids don't like to hear her sing, the cads. They outrageously tell her to stop. She doesn't listen to the charts any more either. (Sorry ... Amy who?)

6.i) This woman gets attached to things like her hot desk, her business card, her preferred parking spot.

6.ii) This woman keeps silly things like outgrown baby socks, pieces of art which should by rights have been filed In the Bin, miswritten shopping lists and protestations of love ...

To Mummy
I hope yoe have a smashin Morthers Day
Have a niese day
extamanayt Darlix
Love Jack
XXxxX I love yoe

. . .

This little woman went to work
This little woman stayed at home
This little woman pureed roast beef
This little woman had a son (and then another, and then another)
This little woman went weeeeeeee all the way home, and stayed there. For quite some time. And found in the end, it wasn't too dissimilar from being at work. Only different.

It is early March already. We are on the M40 to Claudia's house and the inaugural old friends' Baby Viewing Party. Claudia is my old flatmate from university. As are Doctor Pip and Charlotte Gotta-a-Lot who will be meeting us there with their respective other halves. The other Charlotte was always better off in the chest department than me. For my part, I was once Charlotte Wotta Bot. Alas how times change.

We met at Freshers' week and ended up sharing a house along with five others in our second year. Fittingly, for a houseful of students all squeezed companionably together under one roof, our house was located on Sandwich Street. We shared a love of Abba, the odd pint of cider and greasy take-outs from the Leigh Street chippy. We danced at the nearby halls of residence discos where Salt 'n Pepa agreed to Talk rather a lot About Sex. We thumbed through Cas Clarke 'foolproof' student recipes and ate pasta bakes, occasionally a little more al dente than even an Italian would think wise. Together we sang all the words to 'Dancing Queen', we ate crunchy fusilli, and we formed a bond that's stood the test of time.

Some of us are now married. Some are not. Some continue to drink cider. Some decidedly do not. Some have decided that babies R Us. Some, for the present at least, have not.

Chloe Charlotte is of course delightful. Though slightly scary. Not sure how many of us have held a baby before. With the exception of Dr Pip who delivered babies as part of her training and indeed promised to deliver mine for me at the end of my wedding day, one or two glasses of Pouilly-Fumé later. Needless to say, I am not planning to take her up on the offer.

'So Charlotte, it's your turn next then. How do you think yours will turn out?'

'Hope you shoehorn a Charlotte into the name somewhere at least?'

'Not if it's a boy. Which it will be.' (This from Andrew who professes to be able to predict the sex of all unborn bumps. Interestingly he declared me a boy factory right from the very start.)

'Why not? We're very progressive on names these days?'

47

I wonder though. I wonder what sort of a child I'll have. All of a sudden I imagine a small kid in red Wellington boots and bobbled tights. Boy or girl. We can be progressive on tights these days.

I feel a warm glow for my welly-booted offspring. I like it. That feeling. I spend so much of my pregnancy worrying that sometimes I forget to feel tender.

It's like a marble. There's a delicate twirl of blue in the middle, a precious and wondrous thing. But it's surrounded by a sphere of toughened glass. I know there's a prize lying, beautiful, within. But some days I just can't seem to get to it.

Chapter 4

It is March. I'm about sixteen weeks pregnant. I'm dressed in (elasticated) shorts and sitting expectantly on a plastic white chair in the departure lounge at Heathrow. I feel good. Who can fail to feel good at the airport? (Except when you work for an airline and are drafted in at times of unrest to help field angry passengers and have, unbeknownst to you, 'abuse me' tattooed on your forehead.)

I'd bought the maternity swimsuit. I'd consulted the doctor and snapped up a pair of DVT tights. And I'd packed the suitcases, and then repacked them before they were finally forced shut with the help of a bit of brute force and gravity. Like a large, pregnant woman sitting on top of them.

We'd got up startlingly early (amazing how this pregnancy lethargy can be nimbly shrugged off when there's a holiday to be had) and wended our way to the airport full of anticipation. This will be our last far-flung holiday for quite some time, so, by George, we're going to enjoy it.

I've packed a billion books and, of course, The Notes which *must* accompany me everywhere on pain of a good telling-off from the midwives. But I still can't resist going into WHSmith to pick up a pregnancy glossy. It's busy at work, and the pressure seems even greater what with my forgetful pregnancy brain and tendency to daydream. So with two glorious weeks stretching out ahead of me, I can't wait to get stuck into the manuals and mags. And besides, brandishing this month's *Mother & Baby* on the beach will help make it clear to any doubters that I'm not just fat.

It feels good to actively walk into Smith's and browse the glossies on the pregnancy racks. I can pick them up without compunction. Without a sideways glance. Without needing to sink into my collars like the procurers of mags featuring ladies with no clothes on, which later on would so fascinate my middle-born.

'Mummy, are the ladies hot?'

(Some might say yes, but not in the way you're thinking.)

'Must be, darling. Sweltering.'

There's no secrecy, no smokescreens any more now that I've outed my pregnancy. In fact I want to proclaim it from the rooftops. It was something I chose. I've done my time in the wings, and now I want to crow about it.

Of course, we'd had all the hints and nudges from parents and relations for I don't know how long. 'You've been married quite a while now?' 'I see that friend of yours from school is awaiting the patter ...' and 'I was in John Lewis the other day, idly wandering through the haberdashery department and I simply couldn't help myself stopping to flick through a couple of those knitting-pattern books. Lovely they were. Receiving blankets. Little bootees. Maternity ponchos?' We'd nodded and withdrawn. Not for us yet. Not for seven years after our marriage in fact. Why hurry?

But then we made the decision. One of thousands of little catalysts – active decisions or subconscious actions – that change the course of our lives. Only this was quite a big one, one that may need to clothe itself in a maternity poncho in fact.

I'm seated in the back row. The plane is packed. There's a buzz of contained excitement. An air stewardess is making her way up the aisle. 'Tea or coffee? Tea or coffee? Tea ...' I'm off caffeine at the moment and Dirk soon wishes there was something a little stronger, or smelling salts, perhaps. Clowns to the left of him, jokers to the right, he's sitting with a 'stuck in the middle' frown one along from me. Mindful of my delicate state, he'd manfully offered me the aisle seat. It's a wise move. Although I'm ever needing to go to the loo at the drop of a hat, the DVT tights I'm wearing are so uncomfortable, I still need to keep getting up to ensure my toes don't drop off, which might prove a tad inconvenient.

Trying to take my mind off the toes, I'm flicking thirstily through my new mag like a child with the Christmas Argos catalogue. My eyes are popping. There's an article on motherly guilt – guilt at the drinks you drank, the ciggies you smoked, the sk8ter dude acrobatics you performed in the car park when you slipped on that banana skin of all things – all before you knew you were pregnant. There's an article about pregnancy stuff that your best friend might've failed to mention but which you *definitely* need to know. (Gulp!) And there's an article on food cravings: fact or fiction? (Hmm, I wonder as I look over my shoulder to see if the stewardess has any lip-puckering slices of tart green apples in her trolley.)

I don't know what to read first. I wonder briefly if it's possible to scan a page and read two articles at once. Like reading piano music. Opening an experimental page I alight upon a woman embarking on a water birth teamed up across the staples with an article on 'cures' for morning sickness. In one, slightly rich sensory glance, I take in an oversized paddling pool wrapped in clingfilm, the smell of coffee, a silent but graphic groan, the whiff of strong perfume, water tinged scarlet and a steaming plate of Chicken Tikka Masala. Hmm. On second thoughts, perhaps this blend-reading lark mightn't catch on.

I turn my attentions solely to Mrs Waterbirth. Oh my, yes that one *is* stomach-churning. And in Technicolor, too. I sneak a furtive glance around the cabin to check the stewardess, green apples or no, is still at a safe distance and that my neighbour across the aisle is thoroughly engrossed elsewhere. I feel like you do on the Tube when you're reading a perfectly innocent book and then all of a sudden a saucy bit jumps out at you from the page. You blush, round your shoulders, quite sure that your fellow passengers can see right through the cover of the book you're using to shield your face and have you down as a confirmed pervert. Guilty as charged!

'What's *that* you're looking at?' asks Dirk with undisguised disgust.

'It's OK, I'm not a pervert,' I almost blurt. Instead I say nothing, round my shoulders a little and play hard to get.

What should I say? 'That'll be us in the not too distant future, love' or 'Did no one say there might be blood?' or 'You can't really imagine Liz Hurley looking like that can you ... well, maybe not quite like *that*.'

Before I decide on my retort, however, I'm stopped in my tracks.

'Dirk?'

His eyes have rolled heavenward and his head has lolled back. Is he play-acting?

'Dirk? What's wrong? Dirk!' I jab him fiercely in the ribs. The air hostess bustles up to see what the commotion's all about.

'Ugh,' he stammers, 'I'm OK, I think. Just not very ... ugh ... good with blood, that's all. Can I have some water?'

'You had me worried there,' I say to Dirk when coffee-or-tea woman rushes off to get some bottled water.

'Me too,' says Dirk. 'I thought for a minute you were going to insist that I attend the birth.'

I'm not saying that Dirk's a traditionalist. But the idea of him *not* attending the birth would fit.

He plays chess. He listens to Elgar. He hails from the Netherlands, where people ride those quaint sit-up-and-beg bikes and skate across frozen canals like in Olde Worlde Christmas cards. (Though to be fair I can't see him personally sporting a frock coat, a muffler and/or a handlebar moustache.) He asked my dad for my hand in marriage over a pint in The Rocket on the Euston Road. Not exactly in smoking jackets in the library, but not a bad approximation, some might argue, an inn being a popular place of learning extraordinary new things, and this one being a mere stone's throw away from the new British Library.

Dirk would probably *like* to wear a smoking jacket, however, and chew distinguishedly on the stem of an old-fashioned pipe. If he was able to stomach the wares of Messrs Benson & Hedges, perhaps he even would? But with or without Sherlock's preferred accessory, I like to think he can be the quintessential gentleman when he tries. To be smooth and suave and know how to behave in every situation. To hail taxis, open doors and bring flowers from time to time. Oh yes, this one would've ticked all the boxes in a girly magazine quiz.

Has Your Man Got What it Takes to be a True Gent?

Take this sensational etiquette quiz: is your man a gentleman or a cad, a paragon of good manners or a slob, a shining example of manhood or a good-for-nothing waster?! Read each question and tick the answer that most applies! Good luck ... to you, and most importantly, to your other half!

1) Do you tend to find that your man:
   a) Flashes his cash and wears head-to-foot bling?
      or
   b) Goes about in several-years-old Converse baseball boots, preferring not to flaunt his assets?
2) When out in public, does your man:
   a) Pick his nose or stick his little finger in his ear to clear the wax out?
      or
   b) Abstain from openly grooming himself (except when called upon to do his party piece toenail-chewing stunt which is, I know, somewhat questionable)?
3) When it comes to punctuality, is your man:
   a) Ruinously late ('Oh, you meant 10 o'clock *a.m.*?')
      or
   b) Always, in the immortal words of Black Box, 'Ride on Time' which is, obviously, all about a punctual gent in a well-cut suit accessorised with cufflinks, tie bars and an understated yet classic silver timepiece?
4) When he shakes your hand, does your man:
   a) Offer you a limp-wristed clammy palm number?
      or
   b) Get a grip. I'm his wife. We don't do shaking hands.
5) When it comes to speaking, does your man:
   a) Slip into a faux-Caribbean lilt and pepper his phrases with 'respeck's, 'innit's and random 'bo selecta's (whatever that means)?
      or
   b) Say 'I beg your pardon' and 'excuse me' and 'yes, darling, I know you're *always* right'?

If you chose mostly Bs, well *all* Bs in fact, then your man is ... golly ... *my* man! ('Oy, are you looking at my bloke?')

Your true love is stable, dependable and a proper gentleman with old-fashioned values. He is charming and debonair. He is sophisticated masculinity personified. He is David Niven. He is old school Bond. He is Anthony Head with a cup of steaming Gold Blend. He is a perfectly executed LBW followed by cucumber sandwiches in the pavilion. He is not George Clooney in a green smock and latex gloves.

I think that he'd happily shrug on the mantle of the caricature traditionalist dad, pacing up and down outside the delivery room, not risking the sight of blood.

Perhaps I'll need to recruit Mum to come in and hold my hand in labour then? Hospitals are, after all, her domain. She can do blood and antiseptic odours. She's comfortable and confident there. I wonder if she'll fill in the gap should Dirk decide to decline. The thing is, I don't really know as yet. That's the quiz question about which I haven't got a clue.

When it comes to labour day, will your man:

a) Slip confidently with you into the delivery room, cheer at the appropriate spots, squeeze your hand at the appropriate spots, live through it all like a man ... maybe even cut the cord?

or

b) Say 'I beg your pardon' and 'excuse me' and 'I think I just need to go and check the parking meter. Outside. Needs must, you know ... Traffic wardens eh? Sheesh.'

I'm picking my way barefoot along the hot beach. The sand is a breathtaking white. Birds are cawing loudly above. Dirk's walking a few paces ahead of me, our shoes slung over his shoulder. I'm not feeling great. There's a sudden hot rush of blood to my head and I come over all dizzy. I know I should call Dirk over. Instead I just sit.

Realising I'm no longer following him, Dirk spins round and quickly retraces his steps.

'Everything OK?'

'I think so. Just felt a bit dizzy all of a sudden. Bit hot.'

'Revenge for the plane stunt?'

I half-smile back. He really did faint momentarily; I'm just threatening.

'Perhaps we should go and sit in the shade for a bit,' he says, pulling out a bottle of water and handing it to me.

Retreating to the shade sounds good. Feels right just now. Perhaps I need to get used to sitting down a bit more. Look at things from a different perspective. After all, this meandering about in searing temperatures can't be good for you for long. 'Yeah, that'd be great,' I mumble. 'I just felt a bit hot under the collar there for a bit.'

And while the simmering heat continues to beat down, I reflect once again on how things are set to change.

Islington Gazette   A few years hence

FREQUENT FLIER DEVELOPS JET FLAG

Arsenal, London – Looking to save on the rising cost of fuel, BA has just sent out a personal note of congratulations to a former employee who has made a significant personal step towards shrinking her carbon footprint. Mrs Charlotte Moerman, 34, of Highbury, said she felt 'much more grounded' since stopping flying, well, anywhere at all really. Questions are being asked, however, about what ever happened to her itchy feet?

BOOKINGS PLUNGE

In a statement to the press, a spokesperson for HM Passport Control and Customs reported a sudden and complete drop in Mrs Moerman's comings and goings to foreign climes. 'She and her other half just don't do it like they used to,' claimed an insider.

FLIGHTS BOON

Mother-of-three Moerman had always enjoyed a good foreign trip. Her friends and family were initially delighted, therefore, when she scooped a plum job with household name British Airways. Despite regularly jetting off to stunning business-meeting locations such as Dubai, Jo'burg and Newcastle, Moerman, claim friends, didn't lose touch with her roots, regularly booking herself in for a half-head of highlights at Zebra Hair and Beauty on Blackstock Road. Indeed, though Moerman and husband Dirk (40) quickly went on to enjoy numerous holidays using her generous BA staff flight concessions, jetting off at hugely discounted rates to all corners of the globe, they never forgot their family and friends. They frequently brought back gifts of filched BA travel bags, hotel-branded soaps and once, a rather fine fluffy white dressing gown (allegedly).

END OF AN ERA

But somewhere along the line, that all stopped.

Who, now, would procure the little pots of moisturiser

and one of those dinky sewing kits they'd been hinting at for actually quite a while? Disillusioned, the family began to demand an explanation.

CHANGE OF LOOK

And they didn't need to look long. The next time they set eyes on Mrs Moerman, she'd significantly altered her appearance. Gone were the suits, the fistfuls of crisp boarding passes and the neatly packed codjecar. 'These days she looks more like a backpacker,' said our source, who didn't wish to be named for fear of reprisals. 'She looks physically shorter, laden down as she is with all manner of apparently essential crap.' Namely, it seems, a bulging shoulder bag, a child strapped to her front and pushing a buggy that's sagging from the load of two more children, a buggy board, an upturned scooter, three coats, the nappy bag, a selection of snacks in case of sudden famine, half a dozen *empty* raisin packets, the crumpled rain guard, a moth-eaten cuddly toy and an umbrella. Which she never uses because it's not hands-free. 'No wonder she doesn't go abroad any more. They'd never let her on the plane.'

DEFIANT

When our reporters caught up with Mrs Moerman she was sitting on the floor sorting out jumbled puzzle pieces with the help of her trio of strapping lads.

'I tell you, being at home with this lot knocks the spots off jet-fretting around the world. And if the Isle of Wight was good enough for Queen Victoria, it's good enough for me!' she claimed defiantly.

Betraying an underlying undercurrent of dismay,

however, was one of the young Moerman boys. The lad, who cannot be named for legal reasons, seemingly gave voice to an overall feeling of disgruntlement, saying 'I waved at the plane in the sky today, but I didn't see Daddy waving back.'

LAST LAUGH

In a further turn of events, however, it seems that Mrs Moerman is set to get the last laugh. In recognition of her contribution towards reducing gratuitous holiday carbon emissions, she has received a Limited Edition Commemorative Certificate sent personally (yeah, right) from the offices of Willie Walsh CEO, British Airways. Willie, she claims, has also invited her and a guest to pop in for complimentary smoked salmon sandwiches, any time, just call in. Moerman says she's hoping to take her buggy and a passport, just in case she gets lucky and can blag a standby ticket to somewhere hot.

Mr Moerman, it seems, will be on babysitting duty.

I'm reclining lazily on a hired-for-the-day lounger. The trees rustle above my head. The ocean laps gently at the nearby shoreline. I'm reading a Salman Rushdie from a few years back. Since swapping the Tube in favour of a commute by car, my reading has dropped off to staggering-home-in-killer-heels-at-the-end-of-the-night-out slow. I'm no longer up with the latest releases. And in my current torpor, I'm not even keeping up with the old.

I let the book drop closed and look down my recumbent form. There's a burgeoning bump beginning to grow. I think I've felt a few light flutterings but I can't be sure if it was the baby or a little too much 7Up. I wonder when I'll cease to be able to see my toes. I wonder when my toes will next paddle through distant shores. I wonder if I packed the nail clippers. I seem to be wondering rather a lot these days.

Chapter 5

It's a Saturday in early summer. The sky looks a promising blue. Cars and the odd bus zip by, some with undamaged wing mirrors. Dirk's clutching an *A–Z* and I've got half an eye on my watch. We're tramping along Manor Road, on our way to the first of a two-day antenatal course. Dirk's as pleased as Punch was on the day that Political Correctness came to town.

We've lived in Highbury now for about nine months. In the time it takes to gestate a baby we've learned, well, shockingly little about our near neighbourhood. We've tramped up to The Fields and occasionally on to Upper Street. We've bought ourselves ruinously overpriced cheese from the cheese shop. And we've pottered around the streets on a match day, drinking in the carnival atmosphere and the smell of frying burgers.

What we haven't done is explored much further afield. Dirk's more familiar with Changi airport than his own backyard, and I'm back and forth up the M4 like a Heathrow-bound bungee jumper. Aside from the odd sortie to Homebase, once we're back on home territory, the front door swings languorously shut. Well, there's been DIY to do and lately, a bit of obligatory bun-in-the-oven taking it easy, too.

This is less than can be said for the galaxy-trotting former occupant of our home. According to the vendors of our house,

Patrick Stewart had once had a room here. We were never sure if he was responsible for the large London bus wheel that was languishing in the basement upon arrival. A student trophy after a night out ('Shall we take this one Patrick?' 'Make it so'), or an abandoned spare from the Starship *Enterprise*?

My mum is originally from County Durham. When I was small, we'd make the epic journey once or twice a year to visit her parents and siblings who live there still. We'd wend our way from south of London, up the M1 and on towards The North, capitalised as though it were another country.

To a child it seemed an eternity of Little Chef coffee breaks, keep-'em-sweet travel lozenges and I Spy (something that flew past the window five minutes ago). To mark the progress of our journey, we'd feverishly look out for the steaming chimneys at Ferry Bridge, the first sign for Scotch Corner or the lay-bys in which I'd been memorably car sick.

When we at last completed the marathon, we'd all heave a sigh of relief. The car would approach around a blind corner, Dad would honk the horn in triumph, and we'd pull into a vacant spot behind number 12 or just over the road on a hillock outside The Club. Once parked, we'd unfold our cramped limbs, bundle in through the backyard and be enveloped in warm embraces and 'haven't you grown's. We felt wholly welcome. It was good to arrive.

I clutch my hand to my side. A stitch is beginning to nag as if to say 'Why on earth did you walk?' I am beginning to wonder the same myself.

It's a colourful journey as we head into streets unknown on a Saturday morning towards Stamford Hill. Actually, it's more of a black-and-white journey, but interesting nonetheless as the Jewish community makes its way to and from the synagogue.

While they hurry noiselessly on their way, I feel a grumble coming on.

'Are we nearly there?'

'Not far now,' says Dirk in mock parental retort. He's taken control on this one; I'm following limply and not a little hot behind. It's quite calming to be led like a child, allowing him to take charge. I'm the one who needs looking after now, and I'm reasonably content to play follow-my-leader, though a car ride might've been nice. I just wonder as I trail along behind him, thumb stuck into our ancient A–Z, whether to believe his confident bluster.

Fortunately, as it turns out, it's not just a fob-off as we turn right into the tree-lined road we had been aiming for. I feel like honking a horn in triumph. We arrive just in time at the white front door of a tall Victorian house. I have a perpetual fear of being late so I'm pleased to note we've made it with two minutes to spare. Albeit with a stitch and a hint of a cloud across my warm forehead.

I step up to the front door. Dirk shuffles expertly in behind me. There are certain things that are indisputably the department of the missus. Things like remembering the mother-in-law's birthday, ensuring there's always a clean pair of socks in the drawer and, as I'd later discover, paying the babysitter at the end of a night out. (Dad's job is to 'help' play computer games.) Today it's definitely down to me to take the lead. Dirk skulks moodily in the background as I ring the bell. The door is opened. We're ushered in. It appears, naturally, that we are the first.

We are sitting on beanbags in a room at the top of the house. Everyone is shoeless. There are six couples, six large bumps, one five-year-old and our new flexible-looking friend, the antenatal teacher.

The soft furnishings and bare feet are meant, I think, to help us feel relaxed. To be honest, I'm anything but. The teacher looks let-it-all-hang-out relaxed, as though ready to perform a complex yoga position by way of a warm-up. The little boy looks pretty relaxed too as he contentedly empties a bag of toys onto the cushions, oblivious to the electricity in the air around him. And the beanbags are looking very, well, very sort of pouffy.

But everyone else looks a little strung out. There's a lot resting on this class. We're hoping to learn some top tips on dealing with childbirth, and for someone to reassure us that it really doesn't have to hurt *that* much (does it?). We're hoping to make fledgling friendships with those who, by the throw of a dice, are all pregnant at the same time, happen to live nearish by and are ready and willing to use antenatal classes as a kind of new parents' matchmaking service. And we're all hoping our feet don't smell.

Glancing around the room before kick-off, I can't help but feel that we're a cruel parody of a retirement home day room. We're all sitting obediently in a prescribed circle, backs to the wall and looking inwards (some at their newly varicose-veined legs), and all patiently waiting for direction on what happens next. Or at the very least a cup of tea and a biscuit. Unlike our aged friends, however, we're quite literally bursting with life. And there's more on the cards today than a game of draughts or a bit of daytime TV.

It seems a long time since that Christmas Eve meal when I'd been full of doubt and joy and grape juice. I am now well into the thirty weeks. It is the third trimester apparently, but as I'm still unsure if it's 'try'mester or 'tree'mester, I prefer to call it the home straight.

Way back then, I'd mistakenly thought this pregnancy was

all about baby, Daddy and me. But no, I've also worked out there are many, many more people in this relationship than just us three. What with the advice-givers, the 'in my day' teeth-suckers, the bump-patters, the 'any thoughts on names yet?' information-prodders, the it's a boy/it's a girl/it's a baby old wives' tale enthusiasts and the very, very keen grandparents to be, it was always going to seem a little crowded. But get this, here am I actually wanting to bring extra bods into the equation. I'm actively going out in search of new friends. Or even just one.

Forget my blind date with the tot in my tummy, I'm now frantic to match myself with potential friends, confidantes and anyone who can take me through exactly what a TENS machine does just one more time, *very* slowly.

I wasn't quite desperate enough to walk into the room wearing a 'please be my friend' placard round my neck, but I had searched a few websites looking for subtler tips like these:

New Mums Meeting New Mums – Advice & Tips Centre

- You get only one chance to make a first impression. People who smile, wear recently bought clothes that don't gapingly show off your stretch marks and who look (even if they don't feel) reasonably in focus get up to ten times more responses!
- Cast a wide net and kiss a lot of frogs. Widen your search preferences. Subtract a few inches from your preferred girth mate – you won't notice that she's skinnier than you when you're discussing perineum tear stitches.
- Work on your new mummy friendships the way you work on your other projects. Set goals and keep at it. You have to *talk*

to people to hope for any degree of conversation back. Reply to all who address, even if it's just a polite 'Bog off. You look like a weirdo.'

- So many ways to connect, so little time. Try a new communication feature every day. Hang around the nappy aisle in the supermarket one day or sit and wait for a fictitious baby clinic appointment at the GP's – just get a conversation started. You may feel you look a bit desperate. Don't worry, you do.
- Parenting website message boards are where members discuss issues of the day – join in. They can't see that you haven't washed your hair or cleaned your teeth for a fortnight.
- Remember, 'Eighty per cent of success is just showing up.' And not looking/acting like a freak helps.

Internet sites can be so helpful sometimes I find.

I'm sitting crossed-legged on the carpeted floor. I'm not generally a cross-legged kind of a girl. Not least because my knees have an annoying habit of clicking into a locked position like some smart anti-theft device, the release mechanism for which is pretty dodgy at the best of times. And this is not one of the best of them.

The six couples, whose names I've already forgotten, are all unbearably close. Funny, I'd thought that the classes were going to be about 'breathing', advanced Pelvic Floor Exercises and a nice little chat about drugs. I hadn't envisaged covering coping strategies for strangers invading your personal space. But, fair dos, I guess I'll be needing them. Midwives could reasonably be renamed Space Invaders so I'd better learn to loosen up fast.

Luckily, the only person who's actually touched me so far today is the one whom I'm fortunate enough to have known longer than five minutes. The teacher has suggested we try out some massage techniques that might help soothe pain during labour, so Dirk is grudgingly kneading my lower back. Each couple is having a go but looking thoroughly awkward at their task. Unless I'm mistaken, the only one who's feeling soothed right now is the teacher.

Everyone's being very British. Yes, we may have conceived a child together. But surely we're not now going to have to touch in public! Amongst other people touching each other at that! Suddenly it all becomes clear. Although she's cunningly told us this bit's about pain relief during labour, that's nothing but a load of claptrap. This warm-up exercise is in fact a genius way of relaxing us into the session and providing us each with our parental matchmaking chat-up lines.

I see that though our discomfort levels have briefly shot up like a gas ring turned to max, this is all part of the cunning plan. Being good girls and boys, we're all stoically getting on with the job in hand, gritted teeth, forced smiles. And then, lo and behold: a bit of fleeting eye contact, a few shared grimaces and some hammed-up mutual groaning. The antenatal teacher has waved her magic wand and, suddenly, we're as one.

We've found unity by clinging to our Britishness over this rather awkward massaging business. Stoicism and mutual grumbling have bonded us like no dry name-giving introductions could. Now we're on a roll. Someone makes a comment on the weather. Someone else apologises when glancing an accidental elbow into their neighbour. Someone compliments another's magnificent bump to which the other responds self-deprecatingly, 'Oh, that old thing, it's just something I picked up *months* ago now. Yours is better.'

We politely queue when practical materials are handed out to illustrate what happens during labour and birth. We snigger over the hairstyles and fashions to cover our discomfort over the nudity. We groan companionably at the sight of the dummy baby being passed through the dummy mummy and her small surely-it-won't-fit-through-that cervix. We blush when the teacher uses anatomical words that you just don't say out loud in public.

We heave a sigh of relief when it's deemed time for tea.

It is my last day at work before maternity leave kicks in. It's mid-June. The air conditioning's chuntering away, irritating the eyes of contact lens wearers everywhere and boosting the sales of skin moisturising products across the city. It's not helping me much. Feeling large and ungainly, my emotions are pogoing all over the shop and I'm feeling distinctly hot and bothered.

Yet I'm also tickled with a whisker of mad holiday abandon. I'm demob happy. Slightly loopy. I've got myself a large black bin liner and I'm approaching my four-drawer battleship grey filing cabinet with glee. I've got to condense all my clobber into one small drawer before leaving today. After hoarding wads and wads of virtually untouched paperwork for years, I am finally seeing sense and recognising the need to bin the lot.

Oblivious to the everyday goings on all around me, I'm totally focused on the job. There's a film of perspiration across my forehead and I'm glinting with steely determination. I'm spreading my considerable weight across my squared legs. I am Clint Eastwood, alone on a dusty street and braced for some high noon action.

The bulging hanging file I eye up first smoulders back at me as I lick my lips, ready to do my worst. It is the paper trail of some hideous project that I'd gratefully put to bed in the drop folder several months previously, never to see the light of day again. Until now. It is a mean-looking fella. If this file had a name it would be something like Wild Bronco PIR or Spit for short. Spit narrows his eyes back at me, gutsy to the last. I draw. Pause. And then let rip. With a last sigh, and a spunky sounding whoomph, Spit slips resignedly into the black bag and finally hangs up his boots.

He was but the tip of the iceberg. Inside there are, amongst others, Butch Checklist and the SLA Kid, Wyatt Emergency Procedures, Billy the KPIs, Calamity Planes and Associated Corporate Design Guidelines and, last but not least, the Magnificent Seven, a series of boxed business cards, charting my changes in job title. These drawers are Buffalo filled with my potted BA career, a record of time and effort spent. Chiefly flouting the call for a paperless office, it seems.

And as I haul it out and cram it very ungreenly into the bin bag, I wonder what on earth I think I'm doing. This unassuming grey filing cabinet has been a silent but faithful friend. It's stood there unquestioning and solid, a guardian of targets met and approvals given. A guardian of the evidence that attests to the fact that – yes – I've actually achieved a fair bit. In spite of my ricocheting self-esteem, in spite of my dread of public speaking and in spite of my Essex-girl roots – I've ... blimey ... actually managed to do something with myself.

I look down at the heaving black bag at my feet. It's bulging with crushed paper and the plastic is looking a bit thin in places. It's bursting with the paper trail that connects me to what I do. To what I *did*. It's the stuff that bears testament to the person I am, or *have* been, when wearing my professional hat. And now I'm in the process of glibly chucking it away. In one way it's liberating. In another, it's terrifying.

My hands are grubby with ink. The cupboard's nearly bare. I take out the last box of business cards bearing my married name, my soon-to-be-returned mobile number and my soon-to-be-defunct job title. I take one out for keepsake. And then I plop the others in amongst all the rest.

About three years previously, we'd returned to the UK following a couple of years living and working in Paris. I had no job to go to, but I was pleased to be back on home turf.

Some things were unchanged: the weather, obsessive discussion of the weather, and Michel Fish *still* getting it wrong on the telly. But some things were unmistakably new yet in a reassuringly British way.

There was the fanfare over some new satellite technology that was to be used in the annual battle against autumn leaves on the railway lines. There were disgruntled drinkers lamenting the ever-rising price of a pint of real ale, which was now on average a shocking £1.64 a throw. And then there was a newly coined phrase being bandied freely around. PMT – Pre-Millennial Tension – was what stressed Brits were apparently suffering from in the run up to the year 2000. Or Pardon My Trolley, as I preferred to call it, as feverish shoppers stocked up on crates of champagne, party poppers and token tins of baked beans for good measure.

Above and beyond all that, a strange and compelling new beast had come to town. The Triffids had nothing on the all-conquering voracity of this strange new brute. I didn't concern myself outright that it'd cause the breakdown of society or make small children hide in horror – though actually perhaps that's not far off the truth. All I know is that all of a sudden in radio ads, on carrier bags, on massive billboards and yes, on the packaging of those fast-selling cans of beans, *everywhere*, the mighty URLs had stormed civilisation as we'd hitherto known it. The www.phenomenonhadarrived.co.uk.

And so it came to pass that while people were going dotty

over the dot-com sensation, I poised my pen to draw a fresh line in my dot-to-dot career path. After taking in a tutti-frutti mix of student holiday jobs – trashy perfume sales, market research surveying and ... yawn ... database inputting – I'd accumulated a chequered CV which bore testament to my experience in publishing-cum-new media-cum-marketing-cum-jack of all trades and mistress of none.

I'd like to say that I responded to a BA job advert, was successfully shortlisted, knocked 'em for six in my interview and cruised forthwith into a top-dog job. But that would be a pack of lies, and anyway, I don't like to invite canine comparisons.

Instead, I pretty much fell on my feet when I was taken on as a temp and then made permanent in what was then called the Digital Channels team. We began as a team of twelve, which felt a significant number. The commute was crap, the pay wouldn't take your breath away, but it felt good. And so I stayed and I threw myself wholeheartedly into it and worked long, long hours.

This, in case you weren't paying attention earlier, is kind of what I signed up for:

Employer:	British Airways
Reference:	WYSIWYG – i.e., Me
Contact:	Louise, bless her heart, who got me in through the rear doors which are located here, here and here
Location:	London Heathrow – Approximately 35,000 feet from my front door. With clear skies all the way, your journey time today is estimated to be a jolly long one In an emergency, strip lights on the M4

	will guide you all the way to your nearest hot desk
Industry:	Airline – New Media – Old Tricks – New Dogs
Job Title:	Variable – Should be stowed on business cards in your drop-files locker or under the seat in front of you
Contract:	Permanent ... ish
Hours:	Approximately 10.5 hours daily
Salary:	Not high-flying

Now sit back, ensuring your seat is in the fully upright position and your tray is stowed away in the seat back in front of you, and do enjoy your flight.

I'm back at my desk. I've cleared the physical decks. Now comes the emotional bit. I know that they'll start to hover soon so I'd better lick the last of my jobs. I think about what to write for my out of office email: 'Charlotte is currently out of the office on maternity leave. She'll be returning to the office ... well, probably never if she can help it. Oh, don't be daft. Only joking! Perhaps she'll be begging to come back next week anyway, ha, ha, ha.

(Someone remind me to ask about company policy on bringing a squalling, red-faced newborn into the office and begging for life to return to normal. Remind me to check the instructions for the rewind button. Remind me to ... phooo phooo phooo, practise those calming deep breaths for labour every now and again.)

If your query is urgent, please contact somebody entirely different. Charlotte is in the final throes of pregnancy brain. And thereafter it's anybody's guess.'

I've never been particularly good with change. I'd just about mastered francs and centimes then they ditched them for the Euro and now I haven't got a clue. Perhaps it's the fear of bewilderment, of losing control or of feeling that I don't belong. Whatever the case, I simply don't cope well with the prospect of change. I get all worked up. I blow my anxieties out of proportion. I either overeat or starve and I sleep badly. I retreat into my nervous shell and fret.

I went to boarding school when I was twelve. I remember sewing name-tapes into my pristine shop-smelling uniform. I remember packing an enormous charcoal-grey trunk with everything I could possibly need in the coming weeks plus a small and cute fox, my cuddly little bedfriend, whom I'd christened Scamp. And I remember brushing my hair into the tightest of ponytails, what would now be known as a Croydon facelift, and preparing to leave home. I was dressed in the uniform. Pictures were taken. I was nervous. I was goofy. I didn't know what to expect. My throat felt tight and I was stifling the urge to cry. This was it. Big changes were afoot.

We arrived at the school. I remember the acrid smell of floor polish, the foreboding iron bedsteads ranked in straight dormitory lines and I remember having Findus French Bread Pizza for our first evening meal in the enormous dining room. I'd never had it at home before. I could soon see why. Heaps of leftovers were scraped into the big black bins at the exit where we stacked our plates. 'For the pigs', I was told. I wonder how they rated it.

I'd been the only one to arrive in uniform, the new girl who didn't know you all pitched up in scruffs on the first day of term. It was the second year of secondary school. Everyone seemed to know each other already. I felt very alone sitting on my borrowed bed, my new pink duvet cover still crisp with creases where it'd come out of the packaging. I clutched Scamp numbly and waited.

Gradually of course, things picked up. I ventured off the bed. I made some faltering friendships. Bit by bit, I explored the school and its grounds – my new temporary home – and saw what it had to offer.

There was that enormous dining room where I stumbled upon the delights of Arctic roll, orange fried bread and Alpen in packets. There was a sweeping open staircase that led from the ground floor up to the dorms about which we told grim ghost tales of those who'd flung themselves from the top floor. And there was the large room with a highly polished floor and lined with wooden lockers where we went for morning recess. We'd each get a slice of bread – some entrepreneur sold butter and honey from her locker – and wait expectantly for the post. Would today be a lucky day when your name was read out? Letters, sent and received from home and from my brother in a different boarding school, meant the world.

There was an avenue of mature trees that circled the perimeter of the sports fields, the site of our tortuous cross-country runs and a place to dilly-dally on a summer evening with friends and *boys*. There were some sunken rooms, known as 'the res' where we could hang about on wetter evenings after prep. There were old cushions scattered across the floor, some graffiti on the walls and a tired built-in stereo system blasting out our favourite hits again and again and again. We got into the groove a thousand and one times. Yeah, we got to prove that we really liked it quite a lot.

But it wasn't all about misspending time in the company of Madonna, TTD and a-ha. Though, granted, I could've spent my entire time poring over Morten Harkett's cheekbones, there was other more important stuff to study. Like discovering how to entertain ourselves on that bonus day off when school was closed because of the Great Storm of 1987. (Old trees, Victorian slates and a gaggle of exposed children didn't mix well with a gale.) Like working out how to convincingly get our hair into those trendy plastic banana clips. (Short answer: quickly grow a thick and curly eighties mop; long-term answer: don't bother.) Like learning how to fit in.

Not that I was ever part of the 'in' crowd, but I didn't want to be a complete nerd either. So I got myself some stonewashed jeans, I started to wear a bit of make-up, albeit it in unwise electric blue, and I went out with my friend Rebecca to buy our first ever single. (Mel 'n' Kim's 'Respectable'. Not in truth a respectable beginning for a music collection but, hey, it was a start.)

Scamp began to stay longer alone on the bed, my powder-pink duvet cover was replaced by another in trendy primaries and the wall behind my bed head lost the fluffy kitten pics in favour of Emilio Estevez, some naked torsoed Athena bloke and, oops, we're back to Morten again.

'Everything all right, Charlotte?' asks Caryn, whizzing in with a plastic-topped coffee in one hand, an armful of files and a mobile phone in the other.

'Yeah. I think so. Just been doing a bit of spring cleaning, sorting out the emails and stuff.'

'You will write won't you? Let us know how you're getting on.'

'Sure, of course I will. You know me and emails.'

My inbox is permanently overfilled. I have a tendency to write everything down. I'll confirm a conversation on schedules, lay out my bullet-pointed expectations on a job, or have a protracted 'real-time' chat with someone who lives and works in a different time zone. There are people I work with whom I've never met, but we email all the time. There are people who work just across the office whom I seem to email more often than speak to. It's a funny old world.

'Anyway. I'll be seeing *you* later, before you head off,' Caryn says raising her eyebrows meaningfully. 'Don't work too hard now, will you?' she concludes before speeding off to her next appointment, leaving a faint waft of Marlboro Lights in her wake.

I swing back round again to face the screen, smile and shake my head. If I find the time around the baby to write to Caryn and if she finds the time to write to me back around the endless meetings and fag breaks, we'll probably spend longer in each other's virtual company than ever before. It's a big if, though.

I thought I'd be killing time today but I'm still busy rattling away on my keyboard. I don't notice the silent nod from Caryn. I don't notice the down tools and sudden hush. I don't notice the ranks gradually creeping in behind my back until, with a jump, I realise I'm not alone.

Some are standing, some are sitting and some are perched precariously on the desktops. There's an awful lot of them. And I'm in the middle, with a safety belt of distance between me and the concentric circles of folks. I feel like Shaggy finding himself in a tight spot surrounded by a motley circle of monsters. 'Like, Zoinks, Scoob, it looks like we've got company!'

There's Del in the corner smirking, probably at another one of his infamous jokes freshly fired off into our inboxes. Anne, mascaraed eyes fluttering, looks up expectantly, hoping no doubt that they get on with it soon so she can head off and get a fag on. There's Jon, wondering who'll be getting the beers in, it's surely only a matter of time. And then there's Liz, the enviably young placement student. She's grinning from ear to ear. Though years away from bearing kids of her own, so she hopes, she's engaged enthusiastically with my pregnancy right from the moment I divulged it. From marvelling at the size of my bump, quizzing me on what it feels like inside and encouraging me to tell her our nickname for it, she's followed my form all along the way like an avid footie fan. (Apparently *her* nickname in the womb was Snoopy. A cruelty, as it turned out, as Liz claims to suffer from big ears. I haven't personally noticed that they're scribbledy black and floppy so I don't know what she's complaining about.)

Caryn's saying something now but it's going over my head. '... for three years ... Newcastle ... animated orange plasticine; Morph! ... Interactive Channel Guidelines ... *Pop Idol*'s Nicki Chapman ... emergency procedures ... *Reservoir Dogs* on crutches ... baby!'

There's a burst of clapping and some wag, probably Gordon, adds a piercing whistle to the applause. I nod and blush and haul myself reluctantly to my feet. I know I've got to do it but speaking in front of a crowd always gives me the willies.

Flash forward several years and here's Jack, dressed up like a monkey. He's in head-to-food brown, there's the obligatory dressing-gown cord tail, and the name of his character's appliquéd in felt across his chest in case of the slightest doubt. 'Boo' poo pooed the face paint offer however. What could be more appropriate than his own grubby, cheeky-looking face anyway?

This was all bravado before the event mind. Now that the show's about to start and he's standing before a roomful of grown-ups, wriggling younger siblings and assorted hangers-on, maybe he'd be grateful for a bit of slap to hide behind? With a nervous smile and a toe drawing small circles on the school hall floor, he's not exactly king of the swingers now.

But perhaps I judge too soon. The lights go down, the CD soundtrack's activated and the cast of animals jumps into life. All of a sudden, it seems, he doesn't give a monkey's about being up there, in the spotlight, under the scrutiny of a watchful crowd. He knows his moves, he knows his lines, he's good to go. He launches into the familiar 'Jungle Rumble' song and he's off and away. A star in the making.

Like him, I found my missing confidence in the scripts, the costumes and the choreography of plays. Reading from someone else's words, wearing someone else's clothes, slipping into someone else's accent, something I discovered I was good at. It was a way of gaining laughs, asking outright for applause in a very non-British way. It was a great way of overcoming fear. Being someone else.

Wouldn't it be nice to be able to reach for a script or have someone direct your moves or lay out the *right* clothes for you in real life?

I clear my throat. There's a sudden itch at the back of my neck that I'm compelled to scratch. I falter for a bit.

'Um. Unaccustomed as I am ... Well, erm, thanks everyone, thanks, Caryn. Oooh. Now that looks interesting.'

Helen and Claire are advancing from the left with a card and an enormous bag between them. Winnie the Pooh and Piglet are on the front proclaiming my new affinity with all things pre-school. It's laden with baby gifts that I see I'm going to have to open here and now. My hands are shaking, but I manage to tear off the paper with a bit of decorum. I think I manage to make the right moves and say the right things.

It's not a leaving presentation as such of course. It's the start of maternity leave and the expectation is I'll be coming back.

I've no idea if I will, but if my three-hour daily commute from Highbury has anything on the decision, it's looking unlikely.

'Phew,' I gasp at the bottom of the bag. 'I thought I'd be getting an Arsenal Babygro if you had anything to do with it, Nick,' I continue, trying to deflect attention from me to the chap who's bigger on the Gunners than Nick Hornby. *Our* Nick makes some responding quip comparing the size of his belly to mine, there's a ripple of laughter and then everyone disperses.

I'm still a bit red-faced and damp across the forehead. It's a relief to head down into the cool underground car park. What an afternoon. I feel tired, emotional and enormous. I swing the outsize Pooh bag into the boot and squeeze in behind the steering wheel. With my beach-ball tum and stretched-to-the-max top I reckon I must look not a little unlike Pooh myself. 'The more I grow, tiddly-pom, the more my clothes, tiddly-pom, are really growing ... far too tight for comfort.'

Shifting my weight a little, I smile as an image of Pooh hanging tightly onto a large, blue airborne balloon flits through my thoughts: Pooh at the start of another big adventure, free as a bird but with scant control over which way the wind might puff and really only a very vague idea of where he might land. Silly old bear!

Tiddly-pomming to myself, I put the key in the ignition, turn and pull slowly off. I glance in my rear-view mirror and watch my impressive office, the early evening sun reflecting off its windows, disappear round a bend. This is it then. Off we go and into the future. One thing's for sure, it'll definitely be one part orange, assuming the Dutch genes are to assert themselves. And the other part will be either pink or blue. But will it be bright, that's the question?

I squint into the low evening sun and move up a gear.

Chapter 6

Lowering myself smugly onto the park bench, I'm sure I'm grinning like a Cheshire cat. What's there not to smile about? I'm free from the shackles of work – the commute, the meetings, the office politics – free from the constraints of time – my day's here to do with as I wish – and I'm temporarily free of needing to meet anyone's expectations but my own. The sun is beaming and so am I.

Stretching out before me is the open expanse of Highbury Fields. Some might query this under the Trades Description Act (at what point does a patch of grass become a field?), but for one who's spent too long cooped up in a car, a hermetically sealed office and a seriously challenged set of maternity trousers, it's looking pretty expansive to me.

And I'm giving it some serious study. Because today I am Detective Trapper, the guy in those handbooks for junior sleuths that Ed and I used to pore over as kids. Detective Trapper was the one with the petrol-blue mackintosh, turned-up collars and a tilted trilby, which was utterly rubbish at concealing that give-away black moustache. We'd flick through the pages picking up tips on how to crack codes, find clues and secretly observe shifty-looking whistlers lurking on street corners. We'd disguise ourselves with talcum powder as grey-haired old gits with dandruff shoulders. We'd search for fingerprints with paintbrushes and more Johnson & Johnson's finest talc. And we'd sing the Shake 'n' Vac song for extra larks, though strictly speaking that wasn't in the book. (What was that woman on, anyway? Had she been shaking or partaking, that's what we wanted to know?) Our room ended up like a bombsite. Those were the days. Ah, what a blast.

Today I've put wads of cotton wool up my T-shirt and dusted talcum powder in my hair to conceal my true identity. (Or have I?) I'm melting into obscurity on the park bench doing some out-in-the-field observations. Combing the scene for clues and evidence. Trying to work it all out. My mission, and I've chosen to accept it, is simply to watch. I raise my imaginary magnifying glass aloft and decide I'm clearly a born super sleuth. Look, I've found *loads* of loiterers. And I didn't even need Petal the police dog to help me find them.

There are all sorts out there. Not far away, a solitary sunbather reclines lazily on the grass, relaxing to 'A Little Less Conversation' through the privacy of her headphones; joggers puff around in red-faced circuits; a fire-engine crew parks up behind the stationary ice-cream van for Flake 99s and a large dollop of toddler hero-worship; the van itself pulls in a slow but steady trickle of customers, crowing in large handwritten letters 'Forget the rest, wer'e simply the best!' (Best apart from when it comes to points of grammar then.)

And then there are the dog-walkers. They potter endlessly round the park, laden with armfuls of stuff. To be a proper dog-walker, you clearly need paraphernalia: slavered-on tennis balls, discreet plastic sacks, Scooby snacks, a lead (traditionalist or up-to-the-minute extendable one), one of those fluorescent plastic 'go-fetch' lobbing sticks and at least one mutt, sometimes two. Occasionally the owners raise their voices, calling their wards loudly into rein. Every now and then they stop to deal with poo. Not dissimilar from the pram-pushing mob, from what my rudimentary observations can gather.

Because for every dog-owner, keep-fitter, mobile-touting businessman or pimple-faced truant, there seem to be ten women at the helm of a buggy. There are tall ones, short ones, fat ones, thin ones, old ones, young ones, and yes, come to think of it, even the occasional one that looks not a little unlike Neil from *The Young Ones*: lank unwashed hair, spot-stressed skin and pasty pale with exhaustion. I wonder where the glowing, peachy mums I'd seen gracing the pages of the pregnancy mags have gone. Perhaps they're all shopping up Marylebone High Street while their spot-faced, stressed looking nannies walk their offspring in the park?

Shopping. I haven't even seriously started on that front yet. OK, a couple of vests and teeny tiny socks, maybe. But it'd seemed too complacent to invest in the big stuff, all that room-filling, *expensive* nursery clobber too soon, 'just in case'. But now, with only a few weeks to go, maybe I should pull my socks up. Yes, let's forget the living, breathing, capricious and worn-out human baby-walkers, which frankly are a bit off-putting, and turn our minds instead to checking out their pushchairs, doing a bit of Snoop Buggy Bugg.

What would Detective Trapper do now? Ah yes, make a list. Let's see:

- What does the nearest buggy look like?
- Is anything dropping out of the shopping net at the bottom?
- Is it gliding straight or does it have Shopping Trolley Veer?
- How many matching buggies are out doing the rounds?
- What colours does it come in?

Ah yes, shopping. That's more like it. Now breathe. And relax.

I am a mummy. Therefore I shop in a calm and orderly mummy-like way. Or that's what I thought I'd do.

Examples of my mother-of-three shopping:

1) FOOD SHOPPING:
   - Ninety per cent online. Who'd go willingly to a supermarket with a horde of whingingly reluctant and/or mad-keen junior consumers who want to buy everything in the shop – especially teeth-rotting drinks, sweets and comics with a plastic mobile phone on the front that you know will break in five minutes flat but which they absolutely *must* have – anyway?
   - Ten per cent top up as you go. A bag of Coxes here, a block of cheddar there, a couple of vampire capes here, well, they *are* only £2.99 and it *is* Halloween in a month. Now where was I? A flagon of blue milk here, a stack of bagels there, a ... hmm, will they eat this fish if I bung on some cheesy mash ... 'Yes, Sid, yes, we're nearly done.' Perhaps with some peas? 'Sid, lovey, really! Sorry, he's *teething* at the moment ... Sid!!' Right. A carton of Ribena here. A Chupa Chup there. Bob the Builder comic? Bring it on. Peace and shameful quiet. And off to the till.
2) CLOTHES SHOPPING:
   - For me? Ha ha ha.
   - For the boys. Well you can't beat a label. In a bag of hand-me-downs. Still *very* proud of my 'Contrast Stitch Fleece Half Zip in Light Airforce' Boden buy: fifty pence in the Salvation Army shop. Occasional guilty trips to Gap. Always in the sale. Well, except that time I just had to buy new jeans for the boys for Jeans for Genes day and I

couldn't send them to school *not* in jeans or they'd have stuck out.

- For Dirk? Well, the departure lounge has an admirable range of men's outlets I always find.

3) TOYS AND PRESENT-BUYING:

- Gah. I'm such a sucker. Who says September's too early to start thinking about Christmas anyway?

My eyes are watering. Is this usual, I wonder, in Trapper's experience or have I just got talc in my lashes? I'm trying to focus on one buggy or pram at a time, but I just *can't* do it, my head is spinning.

It reminds me of interminable childhood car journeys. Tip-top distraction technique this. Give your kids an Eye-Spy Car Number-plate book. 'Now then, you two, why don't you keep yourselves amused by logging down blurred registration numbers as they zoom past our windows?!' Great plan which might otherwise have been called 'How to Gain Whiplash in Your Kids and Vomit in Your Footwells in Three Easy Steps!' Car travel wasn't my specialist subject. Car travel with an array of letters and numbers swimming before my eyes was quite honestly the pits.

The books weren't a complete write-off, mind. Ed and I took delight in spotting number plates from the relative safety of our living room, kneeling upright on the sofa and looking out over the backrests onto the regular stream of traffic of hurtling up and down Notley Road outside. It didn't take us long to work out that all registration plates included a local area code, and that our area used variants of 'OO'. Those were the days. Hours of fun looking out for the prized POO plates. Priceless.

Not what I had in mind for today though. And I'm getting increasingly disillusioned with buggy-spotting too. ('Too many. Please, no more. Can we stop the car? Quick!') Cripes. I think on balance that selecting a MacClaren or a Graco, a Britax or a Chicco, a three-wheeler or four, a travel system or a two-in-one, a will-it-fit-in-the-boot or not-on-your-nelly-but-it's-how-it-looks-that-counts; that can all be Dad's bag. After all, you've got to let them feel involved in the pregnancy eh?

'Is there anything I can do to help, darling?'

'Well, I guess you could always hold back my hair or run some Mr Muscle round the Armitage Shanks when the Morning Sickness Monster comes out to get me? If you happen to be in the country at the time, of course.'

Dad-to-be shuffles nervously.

'Or you *could* join me in giving up alcohol? A bit of solidarity eh?'

Nervous cough. Time-check on wrist-watch. If has one.

'Or how about having a gander at the Mothercare catalogue? See which one you like. Look, here are the pushchair pages. I was thinking of this one?'

'Ah yes, let's have a look, then.
- Will it make the other daddies in the park look on and lust?
- What sorts of shiny gadgets come with it – alloy wheels, integral subwoofers and speakers (ear jacks provided), portable sat-dad?
- Um, how does it handle in reverse?'

Blimey, perhaps I'm just not cut out for this detective lark. The key to gathering clues is surely all about patience and focus. Carefully gathering the evidence, labelling and bagging it for later. Only I just can't seem to settle. I feel like you do when you meet someone wearing one of those Bauhaus polychromatic patterned ties. The ones designed by the guy who invented Elmer the elephant. You do your best to look him in the eye, but you just can't help getting distracted by the colourful barrage of vertiginous bad taste dangling alarmingly just out of eyeshot.

I try to pull myself together and decide to go back to mummy-spotting. I pick one nearby, briskly pushing along a heavily muffled pram. I can't see the incumbent baby but I can hear it yelling indignantly. The mother, grim expression, seems set on breaking a speed-walking record and quickly pounds out of my range. Slightly perplexed, my gaze transfers instead to another pair of mums, dawdling along at a slower pace and wrapped up almost entirely by their own captivating gossip (J. Lo's going SoLo after a marriage of mere months, Jade's made another *Big Brother* gaffe, their NCT cohort who's ... no! ... pregnant again!). To my untrained eye they appear to be ignoring their meandering young charges almost entirely but maybe I'm missing something.

Not to be misled, I continue to scan the field ready to take a few mental 'how to' notes. There are sighers, smilers, shouters and criers, ignorers, exhorters, chivvyers and hippies. There are hand-holders and reiners, shooers and draggers, perambulating joggers and exaggerated praisers: 'Well done, it *is* a lellow car! Who's a clever boy then?' (Lellow?) I feel overwhelmed by the sea of different mummies all of whom have different parenting approaches but the majority of whom seemed firmly and confidently in control. Gulp. This, in the not-too-distant and frighteningly fast-approaching future is going to be me. Yikes.

Feeling like a Brit abroad surrounded by a flood of foreign voices, I reach nervously into my bag for a handy map or a *Time Out* guide. Anything to help steady the nerves and make as though I'm fully on top of things. 'Shortest way to the Louvre? Yes, *bien sûr*, I think you'll find you just jump on the *Métro*, change at *Châtelet* where you'll find half the carriage gets off too. Then you merge seamlessly into the throng, adopt the appearance of knowing where you're going and .... Bob's your *Oncle* ... you'll be just fine!'

Having failed to pack my Paris travel guide, however, I instead dig out a piece of paper and a pen. When the going gets tough, the guff gets going. Usually courtesy of my Bic biro. And so I proceed to assuage my nerves in the way I know best; writing long and effusive letters to family and friends. You can't beat getting out a pen and spidering words across a page. I'm a bit rusty after spending too long at a keyboard, but I find it a pleasure nonetheless. Especially without having demanding emails bursting in on me every few minutes. My fears are pushed under the carpet and I rejoice in a half-cup *full* of raspberry leaf tea kind of way. (Unpalatable though the thought of that might admittedly be.)

Letters finished – well, why exert yourself on a sunny summer's day when you're young, free and mingling surreptitiously with your soon-to-be mates – and I look up, satisfied from my labours. My eyes take a moment to adjust to the glare and then I lazily continue with the people-watching. Forget Trapper, now I just want to watch for the nosy pleasure of it all.

Coursing back and forth through this attractive, but let's face it, trumped-up corridor, go the great and good of Highbury. Though a fair few stop and linger, the majority of these folk are purposefully striding in and quickly out, using the Fields as an easy-on-the-eye throughway between the shops and homes of Highbury and the buzz, hubbub and clipboard-wielding Oxfam reps on Highbury Corner.

Bordering their route is a long terrace of majestic Georgian houses which have silently watched the passing generations of mothers, nannies and miscellaneous others en route from one place to another. They're beautiful, imposing and incredibly desirable (the houses, not the people, although I can't speak for all).

And now I think it is time I join the corridor-wanderers

myself. I gather up my disarrayed papers, stash them into my bag and stride purposefully off. Well, as purposefully as you can manage in my condition.

It's a Tuesday morning. I'm home alone in our bedroom. A worn blue holdall lies open on the duvet. It's seen a bit of action this bag. It was originally Dirk's. Brought it over from the Netherlands stuffed with his chattels when he first came across. It's weathered an English Channel ferry crossing, a slog in a National Express to Victoria Coach Station and quite a few bumpy road and rail trips here and there ever since. It's been about a bit, this old bag.

Dirk of course now has a much smarter wheeled suitcase to take on his business trips, so I've purloined it. I like it. It's a bit thin in places and the zip will need replacing soon, but I'll have it done. Properly. Take it to the cleaners and have it repaired for more than the cost of a new one.

If it ever gets lost, here are the details which I'll post for a handsome reward:

LOST! Brandless Blue Bag

Made in: no idea (label gone, if ever there was one).
Material: One hundred per cent cotton, am fairly sure. Unlined. Faded blue with green handles.
Special Features: Erm, it holds your stuff. (Anti-bacterial microfibre pockets are for wimps.)
Strap: Yep. There is one. Don't think it's detachable, mind.
Volume: Big. But not crazily so.
Last Seen: Under my bed where the dust balls gather.
Reward: A packet of Smarties. (As you can see, it's a much-loved friend.)

I plonk myself down on the bed next to it and tick myself off. It's still only half packed. I'm side-tracking. I need to focus on the job. Why is it that now I've stopped work and I have deliciously all the time in the world, I seem to take five times as long to do anything?

I roll over and tuck in my legs, careful not to squash the contents of my bump. Would it be scandalous to have a little siesta? At half past ten in the morning? I could just lie for a while, I suppose, and muse. Everyone's been telling me to take it easy. All too soon I'll be dragged from my bed by hungry wails, nightmarish shrieks and the cold blast of an errant duvet accompanied by the impish giggles of a guilty sheets thief.

I feel anchored on this bed and that's a good feeling to have. Amidst the whirlwind of physical appointments and fanciful flights of thought, it's good to dally a while enjoying the here and now. Let's just take five and ignore the job that's calling me in. Let's just linger a while and give myself a sense of well-being over all the stuff I've already done in preparation for becoming a mum.

Mum-in-training. To do list:

1) Set out cot that Dirk, his sister and her little girls have all slept, dreamed and dribbled in. Tick.
2) Flick feverishly through the baby names book, making long lists and shortlists and back-of-receipt scrawls when the inspiration strikes. Tick.
3) Pledge my surfaces till they gleam, luxuriating in the novelty of this nesting-instinct thing. (Can I tick if it only lasted half an hour?)
4) Buy packet of Bisto mix. Consider coiffing barnet into seventies 'do. Give the wooden spoon a good hard stare. I

will learn how to peel, chop and baste. I *will* dish up a traditional roast with perfectly turned-out Yorkshires on the side. I just haven't done it yet. Hmm, that'll be a cross then ...

5) Study the ad-perfect mummies and resist disdainful sucking of teeth. Take note of their spotless homes, whiter-than-white whites, germ-free kids with contentedly replete stomachs. Resolve to be just like them, all confident and hygienic in the right places. Wonder if could also be just like that Eva Herzigova in the other ads, but decide not. Best keep it real eh?

I sigh, roll back over and sit upright. So much for enjoying the here and now and reminding myself what I've managed to achieve. I've slipped back off into fantasy land and if I don't get a move on I'll be saying 'Hello Boys' whilst still woefully under-prepared. And I'm not talking going out with, whoops, only my underwear on. (Easy mistake to make when you look *that* good in your bra I guess.)

Right. I *must* pack my hospital bag. I *must* pack my hospital bag. I *must* pack my hospital bag. I just wish it wasn't so off-putting. When I glance through the 'What to pack for hospital' list, I blanch and wish I could disappear back into fantasy land for just a little longer. And perhaps, yes, even back into a dull and predictable team meeting. 'AOB?' 'Erm, yes. Can I (grovel, grovel) come back, tail between my legs and be part of your club again? Please?'

For the labour: snacks, a big T-shirt you don't mind chucking afterwards and a pair of socks. Doesn't paint a pretty picture, does it? Me in a clapped-out T-shirt, clutching a Mars bar with little more than a pair of woolly socks for below-waist-level comfort. Camera (camera?), huge paper pants that even Bridget

Jones couldn't carry off, and sanitary towels, each the size of a Magnum.

I can't feel myself being sold.

You'd think by the time I got to packing my labour bag I'd have had it sussed. Packing and unpacking is the story of my life. The charcoal-grey school trunk, the sit-on holiday suitcases, the business codjecars. Hospital bag? Piece of cake.

I'd got the school packing down to a T by the end. First in, the uniform, ironed if from home, somewhat scrunched if from school. Then the undies, the tights and the socks. The bedding, the towels, the hairdryer, the Walkman, the cassettes ... then Scamp, if I could squeeze him in.

You could tell I was a Brownie by training. 'Be prepared.' That was me. If only the zeal could've lasted me the course. Perhaps I should've just grasped hold of the 'What to pack for hospital' list, made myself a plan and set a deadline; given myself the mental promise of a badge (a cup-of-tea-and-a-biscuit-shaped one) and ensured I washed up and reported to Brown Owl at the end.

Come to think of it, with the benefit of hindsight, maybe this could be the way forward for effective mothering in the twenty-first century. That Baden-Powell was maybe onto something. Modern mums take note. What he did for Boy Scouts in the early twentieth century, perhaps we could do for Mum Doubters a hundred years on.

What's in Guiding to attract a little girl anyway? A safe space, apparently, in which to explore activities, issues and possibilities available to them today. A place in which to undertake new challenges, build up self-confidence and acquire recognition for new skills learned. In which to become skilled at thinking on your feet and feel self-assured you've made the right decisions. To undertake teamwork and acquire leadership skills. To acquire self-awareness and self-respect. To be recognised for doing your best. But hang on, that's what I want too.

I want all of the above, and I'm sure I'm not alone amongst mums. I want to sit in a draughty community hall and pal up with a gang of other stumbling-in-the-dark mummies. (We're all in this together, girls.) I want someone to show me the ropes, let me try it all out in a 'safe space' and give me an award ceremony at the end or at the very least a toasted marshmallow to show I've done it right.

I want the following badges to sew onto my coat-sleeve:

- 'Book lover' – for remembering a list of at least four non-child-related books you've read and enjoyed in the last six years. For buying and stacking at least nine childcare advice books per child. (Reading of these optional.)
- 'Traditional skills' – for preparing packed lunches, sewing on buttons, hemming up trousers, ironing school clothes and tying knots. Usually in self whilst trying to complete arms-length list of 'to do's before pow-wow time.
- 'Agility' – for following a training circuit to school, playgroup and back again, pushing bikes, carrying book bags and spinning plates all the way.
- 'Circus performer' – for juggling. A lot. Oh and tripping, *at the same time*, over the bike stabilisers, the abandoned shoe, and/or Buzz Lightyear, falling in a heap on the floor with an armful of book bags and a cheeky honk of the hooter. Ha ha. Really funny. Mummy got hurt.

I want and deserve all of these badges. And I want a pat on the back and a round of hearty 'well done's for living by the simple but admirable code: the Mummy Tried Law.

On the subject of Magnums and marshmallows, Dirk is keen to

point out at any given opportunity that I need to pack snacks for him too. I'm a bit stuck on this one. I'm keen to get it right. So far I've whittled it down to one or two choice treats. There's a packet of Polo mints. (Can't go wrong with a Polo in your mouth when you're under pressure. Just ask Gordon Brown.) There's a Pot Noodle, my thinking being if Dirk can't stand the heat, he can get out of the delivery room. 'Going to find the kettle' could be our own secret euphemism to save his blushes before the midwives. He'll also need hot water for the raspberry-leaf teabags I've supplied. When things get bad for me, I can distract myself with the sweet revenge of watching *him* drink a cupful of that disgusting stuff because I'll have had enough by then, thank you very much.

Hmm. Not sure this is proceeding in the correct spirit. Don't know why I'm bothering anyway, I still don't know if he'll actually be there or if I'll have to draft in Mum at the eleventh hour. I'm not really fussed if he opts out – I'd rather be the one who's laid back on the bed than him flat out on the delivery room floor. But it'd be nice to know in advance though. Everything's uncertain enough without not knowing who the main cast for the day is going to be. And I'm certainly not packing Pot Noodles for my own consumption.

'You look ready to pop any moment!' says a passing comedian.

Haven't heard that one before. Not.

In truth though, I *do* rather feel rather like a bottle of shaken-up fizz, ready to explode without a moment's notice. I'm walking past Londis and catch a sidelong glimpse of myself in the window. I glance hastily away but too late, the idea's already germinated. I realise I look precisely and unflatteringly like a large bottle of Perrier. I'm the same distinctive shape – bulbous from the neck down – I've a good solid bottom and I'm prone to turning green when I consider what lies ahead. As it turns out, I'm also learning to savour the joys of 'hints-of'.

The automatic doors sweep open and I go in. I need toothpaste for my hospital bag. I shuffle past the ice-cream freezer and on towards Personal Hygiene. Crest, no. Aquafresh, no. Ah, Macleans, yes. I reach for the familiar blue box and look up, inadvertently catching the eye of another woman shopping nearby. She smiles at me. I smile vaguely back wondering, do I know you? I don't *think* so. I head to the till and look shiftily back over my shoulder just in case my new friend's stalking me. It seems not. She's now entirely wrapped up in the Cold Dips and Delicatessen fridge. I've been passed over, utterly forgotten in favour of the hummus.

I leave Londis and zip over to Gregg's. And here we go again. There's a mum buying a bag of doughnuts that she stashes in the bowels of her buggy before ... there it is ... a flash of a smile aimed indisputably at yours truly standing behind her in the queue. Here's another one, slipping an envelope in the postbox with the help of a tottering, tiptoeing two-year-old and ... got it ... a sideways twinkle at me and my bump.

Slowly it dawns on me. I am on the brink of a new club. I feel like Harry gaining an insight into the wizarding world that has always existed alongside his Muggle one but into which he's only just been invited. Conspiratorial little nods and smiles are bestowed quietly upon me as I go about my business. It's not loud, it's not accompanied by any special magic, but it is wholeheartedly welcome. (Thank you and apologies for ever doubting your integrity, Toothpaste Woman.)

Given the choice, I'm more of a P-P-Pick up a Penguin girl than a Club one. There's something so endearingly simple about waddling penguins don't you find? But being part of a club was always good for me. Especially ones with rules and clear entry requirements. Obviously being pregnant and having babies means I immediately qualify to belong in the Mummy Club. But boy, are there all sorts of unwritten rules and hurdles that make it a slippery minefield.

If only it was predictable and safe, like those brainwashing ads of old. You knew where you were with 'If you like a lot of chocolate on your biscuit join our Club' or 'A finger of Fudge is just enough to give your kids a treat' or 'Um Bongo Um Bongo they drink it in the Congo'. If only learning to become a mum was as easy as parroting off a catchy and predictable ditty that everyone else knew too.

Don't think I'm spending all my time casting aspersions on the well-meaning shoppers of Highbury. Sometimes I get to shop further afield too. Oxford Street. Buses and taxis, tourists and tat-stalls flogging Tower Bridge snow globes and faux chef's hats with BBQ King emblazoned across the top. I'm out in the throngs, indulging in some light baby-clothes shopping. Not at the stalls though. Polyester 'I love London' bibs might suit some, but I can't bring myself to love them personally.

I'm heading into John Lewis. It's a rite of passage, I'm sure, to oooh and aaaah over the teeny tiny stuff on the racks here. This is both an excitement and a novelty to me who, even when not transporting around a near-term baby, associated tissue and fluids, and the result of too many Maltesers* these last eight

---

* Re the Maltesers, yeah I know, I know, it wasn't meant to be about eating for two and all that. But it wouldn't be right not to adopt a pregnancy craving and if you're going to do it, you might as well choose a good one. Strangely, even though they're 'lighter than ordinary chocolate' (oh yeah, so what exactly are they then?), I don't look set to emerge from proceedings like a light-as-honeycomb-centred Royal Ballet waiflet. 'Chocolate before the delivery room performance?!' 'Oh, go on, then, if you insist, pass me another one then.'

months, hasn't had the pleasure of going for the smaller sizes in clothing in quite a number of years.

I'm enjoying the shopping trip all the more as Mum's skipping a day's work to tag along. Not for years have we done a double-act splurge on Oxford Street. We'd arrive wide-eyed at Liverpool Street and hit the Tube. Mum ritually grumbled at the noise, the people and the dirt, I'd look out for mice under the tracks and we'd squeeze onto the Central Line tube, all tight handholds and fervent anticipation. We'd traipse for miles, stop at Cranks for the salad bar or soup, and try on endless garments which I'd enthusiastically entreat Mum to buy, or frown at with theatrical repugnance. Think Laura Ashley smocking dresses for the verging-on-teen me. Um, no, Mum.

Treasured times. Bonding in Bond Street. Liberty for two and buttered scones on Regent Street. Wondering if Selfridges up at Marble Arch really did sell fridges. I never questioned whether I'd one day do the same with a daughter of my own. I took it as a given.

What are little boys made of?
Ships and rails and cat-o-nine-tails
That's what little boys are made of.
What are little girls made of?
Mango and Reiss and shoes from Office
That's what little girls are made of.

I've been thoroughly looking forward to this nursery-shopping expedition. For sure, Dirk and I have had a browse together when he happened to be around and could find no reasonable excuse not to. But he doesn't seem at ease wandering round these places as a couple with an invisible placard: 'Look: us and our bump!' Like the betrothed pairs meandering about with their Wedding List clipboards. Or anoraked trainspotters shuffling up the platform, pen and paper in hand, out in a public place amongst normal people, and women. A bit awkward. A bit under the spotlight. A bit frazzled by the whole experience.

Today with Mum is different. United we stand. We are ready, willing and able to fully enjoy our fling with the nursery bling – baby gyms, mobiles, bouncy chairs. Let me at 'em! Not least because, with impeccable timing, we've happened upon the summer sales. What luck, I think, imagining knocked-down birthday presents for years to come.

I look at Mum, and she looks at me.

'Let the games begin!'

And we're off.

There are trays and trays of cutie summer baby-wear at our fingertips and I'm dying to launch into the fray. I must remember my list, however, and not get carried away.

Claudia, very experienced now in these matters, had pointed me towards the source of my list. Chloe Charlotte is now all of five months. Claudia knows what she's doing, I thought, so I bought the book by someone I'd not yet heard of who went by the name of Gina Ford. And sure enough, hurrah, there was a clothes list of what to stock up on for your new baby, and this was it:

Vests	6–8	Socks	2–3 pairs
Nightdresses or sleepsuits	4–6	Hats	2
Day outfits	4–6	Mittens	2 pairs
Cardigans	2–3	Shawl	3
Snowsuit for a winter baby	1	Jacket	1

I take out my crumpled copy of the list. Call me new-fangled, but I can't see how a baby could ever need three shawls. And why eight vests but only two socks? But who am I anyway?

I scan it again, make a mental note to think mittens and pop it promptly back into my handbag to be utterly forgotten from that moment forth.

'Ooh, Mum. Look at this!' (Gingham ribbon-strapped sundress.)

'Oh *yes*. And how about this? Isn't it *gorgeous*?' (Pink polka dot bloomers.)

'Isn't it. What about this one?' (Floral floppy sunhat.)

Unable to resist a bargain, I'm on the verge of scooping up a candy-pink smocking gypsy top in 0–3 months but then the sensible gene kicks in. If I buy something so obviously girly my bump will naturally materialise into a boy. I have no preference one way or the other, but it'd just be daft spending money on something that I couldn't put on a boy without causing him long-term damage should word or photographic evidence get out in years to come.

'Oh go on. It's irresistible. And it's fifty per cent off!' says Mum in an echo of pre-teen me urging her to buy this Alexon skirt or that Country Casuals top.

'No, I can't. It'd be such a shame if it had to stay in the cupboard unused,' I say, placing it back in the tangled pile.

'Your choice,' she replies, which makes me even more firmly resolved to play it sensible as I head over to look at seven prudent white vests. Before getting sidetracked by an adorable newborn swimsuit. (Cross-over straps, ruched top and with a tiny daisy embroidered just above the leg holes.)

By the end of the day, I'm nowhere near the forgotten list of requirements lying undisturbed in my handbag. But, like school uniform lists, surely they're there to be stretched? Which is what I'm feeling like. Stretched. And not a little swollen, which is more than can be said for my wallet.

It's been a good day. I'm now the proud owner of a large pile of neutral newborn clobber. All I need now is the baby.

I am now thirty-seven weeks pregnant. I am, not to put too fine a point on it, huge. I would like to think that I am blossoming. The way you're supposed to when you're pregnant. Radiant in the joy of being ripe as a peach and glowing in the anticipation of imminent motherhood. Alas, I am none of these things.

So what am I like? In my time, I've been variously likened to Corrie's Gail Tilsley, Baby Spice and my brother Ed. For myself, I can only see the likeness between myself and one of the above and he shall remain nameless. That's not to say I wasn't chuffed with the Emma Bunton comparison. Admittedly the originator of this comment was a little tiddly at the time and/or in serious need of her glasses but I rather enjoyed the fantasy of it so I'm choosing to overlook those details.

Besides, there's something deliciously ironic about being compared to the woman who was … a bit weird, didn't you always think … supposed to be a baby while I'm carrying one rather prominently in my belly. At this stage though, I'm very far indeed from any pretensions of Spice Girl glamour – though I'd wear bunches if I thought it might help – and the idea of daring to hope someone might actually wanna be my lover is risible. Right now even my husband is looking at me with thinly veiled horror.

I am huge, I am frequently hot and sweaty, this being a rare blistering summer akin to those of my childhood the likes of which we haven't seen since, and there are rings under my eyes from where Nature plays that cruel trick of sleep deprivation before the baby's even arrived – pre-term acclimatisation to broken nights with frequent nocturnal toilet trips and a frustrating inability to get comfy in bed. Counting sheep doesn't help. Counting disposable paper pants only makes things worse (I've tried).

On top of all that I'm now spending an inordinate amount of time on all fours with my bottom in the air trying rather awkwardly to watch TV while the blood rushes dizzyingly to my head. Once in a while, this improves the viewing experience – I rather prefer Anne Robinson upside down and watching the Aussie soaps this way seems far more authentic. The novelty soon starts to wear though (oh for the days of sitting sedately at a desk!), along with my resolution to turn my breech baby around with the help of gravity. At length I decide to stuff that for a game of soldiers – that's the technical term for reverting to plan B.

Plan B involves travelling down to the maternity wing of the hospital, my labour-bag all packed and going nil-by-mouth for the morning. This could be it ... or it could be just a storm in an NHS disposable plastic cup. The plan is for the doctor to perform an ECV which supposedly stands for External Cephalic Version but in my opinion is surely an acronym for Excruciating Condoned Violence.

It all seems dreadfully nice at first. The midwife gives her name and chats amiably about the weather. The room we're shown into is pleasantly cool with the windows – one-way frosted, I trust – slightly ajar allowing for a refreshing throughput of air. There's a bed for me – thanks – and a chair for him. I try to ignore everything else in the room. If I don't look at the stirrups, then maybe they do not exist.

The doctor strides in. He is calm, efficient and informative. My mouth is as dry as a peanut butter sandwich. I'm not interested in his bedside manner. My eyes are glued instead to his hands. I wonder what he's going to do with them. And where.

Wouldn't it be nice, I think, if the tension – poof – dissolved and they advanced forthwith into a warm and friendly handshake, their owner blustering cordially, 'Congratulations, Mrs Moerman, seems like your lucky day. Sister tells me the scan shows baby *is* the right way round after all. Big mistake! Off you go home now,' and sends me packing. Sadly, this is not what happens.

I've had some relaxant drugs so my eyebrows only shoot up to about hairline level when the doctor commences his attempt to externally (phew) turn the baby round using those hands of his and a bit of light brute force. There's a small chance I might go into labour, apparently, or even need an emergency C-Section, hence the packed bag and breakfast embargo. There's also a rather larger chance I'll soon get off the bed and stage a walk out. It bloody hurts. But then again I haven't been through labour yet so I guess it's all relative.

Dirk holds my hand and gives off encouraging vibes. This is how fans must look on the terraces when they're willing Thierry Henry to pull a winning goal out of the bag but can't physically do anything to help. They can, and do of course shout obscenities when he *fails* to deliver, but I'm hoping Dirk holds his tongue on the performance of the doctor and/or the football-sized star at the centre of the action. At least if you're going to chant, make it positive, I beg silently. On the whole, 'You're shit and you know you are' probably won't go down very well but you *could* always try 'Ooh, Ahh, Can Doct-Ah!'

'Ooh.' (I suck on my teeth.) 'Ahh.'

The hand-grip tightens with every flinch, but Dirk bites his tongue and remains stoically motionless by my side. As does the baby, who's not having any of it. After three or four attempts, we've got no further and the crowd is getting restless.

'Looks like little one's refusing to play ball,' mutters the doctor.

It seems the more he digs the heels of his hands Right Up My ribcage, the more the baby watches and learns. What a great idea! I know, I'll dig my own little pint-sized heels firmly in too!

Eventually, the whistle is blown. Feeling desperately anti-climactic, I wonder if we're allowed injury time as I rub my sore, steamrollered skin. Talk about a turnaround. The woman who wanted to be sent packing is now keen to sign up for more of the action. But no. That's it. Game over.

Sigh. It's a miserable midweek nil–nil draw. Rubbish. Everyone's disappointed. The doc removes his pungent rubber gloves and desists from trying to crack my ribcage. The midwife unstraps the monitors and returns to her paperwork. I swing my legs off the bed and shuffle off out the door, Dirk a couple of paces behind me with the bag.

'I guess it's all still to play for then?' he says as we clasp hands and make our way to the lift.

'I guess it is.'

The lift pings open, we descend to ground, sign ourselves out and emerge, as though from a matinee performance, into the broad light of day.

Chapter 7

It's a Thursday morning. Early. We're walking past the Jeremy Bentham pub. At thirty-eight weeks, I'm feeling as stuffed and pasty-faced as our venerable friend whose 'Auto icon' (which sounds like something technical for your car but is actually the preserved body of Bentham himself) is sitting not so very far away from this place.

I don't know as much as I should about Bentham and utilitarianism, but he doesn't strike me as the sort of fella who'd have misspent his free time boozing down the local. So the naming of this inn, which lies in the shadow of University College Hospital, seems a curious choice. Still, it's a pub that's doing the greatest good to the greatest number of jubilant new dads keen to wet their babies' heads, and you can't say fairer than that.

I squeeze Dirk's hand a little tighter, the nearest soon-to-be new dad in the vicinity. We walk on down the street, him doing the manful thing of steering me gently along as though I've suddenly lost all ability to navigate. (Trust me, I've always been pretty rubbish.)

'All right?' he asks.

'All right,' I echo, having also lost the ability to talk like an individual.

We arrive and walk up the couple of steps into the maternity hospital entrance. It's a funny place. It feels a bit like a museum. I'm waiting for someone to search through the contents of my bag, but no, it's just the usual drill: time and sign your arrival, nod at the security guard and amble on in. This morning the guard nods almost imperceptibly back and yawns. I can sympathise entirely. It feels like the crack of dawn.

At the eleventh hour, everything was turned upside down.

I'd spent the last several months flicking through *What to Expect When You're Expecting* with encouraging pictures of ... yes! ... lots of babies at the back. This forty-week slog *was* going to result in a baby, I tried to remind myself. I looked and looked again at the grainy black-and-white photos the sonographer had packed us off with. I'd watched our junior Olympian kick ripples in my tummy during baths. And I'd looked repeatedly at the *What to Expect* cover-babe with its huge unblinking blue eyes and wondered. It's still not sunk in that I'm having one of these of my own.

What exactly have I been expecting? Well, I guess I'd always expected marriage and kids. I'd have a boy and then a girl, a copy of my own family. We'd live happily ever after in a house in a town with a car and a couple of cats. We'd have a couple of normal jobs, a milkman to deliver our milk, a postman to deliver the post and we'd do just fine thank you very much.

Life would be bright, it would be simple and fun, just as the books had taught us.

It's Maisy's bath time.

She runs the water and puts in some bubbles and in goes duck.

Ding-dong! Oh, that's the doorbell.

Maisy runs downstairs to see who it is.

Oh, it's Tallulah. Sorry Tallulah, Maisy can't come to the door right now. She's busy getting married having 2.4 kids and living happily ever after.

Unfortunately, it's never as simple as that. In the real Maisy book, Tallulah, a bit puzzlingly, barges straight past her betowelled mousey friend, runs up the stairs, strips and gets in the bath too. It's a valuable lesson. Things never turn out quite how you predict. Sometimes you've just got to share the soap. Often with someone or something you were least expecting.

I'd sort of been sidestepping the reality of the baby that was due to arrive at the end of all this, focusing instead on the labour. That's what was coming before the baby arrived, so in my mental 'what to worry about' priority list I put that bit first. I voraciously read the books and mags, I cautiously quizzed my own mum in case she did the dirty and told me *too much*, and I scoured the labour-class photocopied sheets filled with pain-relief techniques, gripping so hard my knuckles turned white. (It hurt a bit when my nails pierced the skin on my palms, too.)

The labour itself became my obsession. That was the bit that I knew would happen first and that I knew I had to face first, before meeting and getting to know my new baby. Only that was the bit that didn't happen at all the way I'd thought it would.

I'd only slept fitfully, in the knowledge that a big day lay ahead. It was like going on holiday, knowing you've got to be up and out at some ungodly hour to check in at the airport. You hardly sleep with the excitement of it all and nerves at missing the alarm call.

After hours of restless tossing and turning, the beep-beep-beep had sounded out loud and queer. 'Wake up! This is it! Rise and shine! It's the day to go and collect your baby!' How weird is that?

It had all been planned. We would go in by Tube. No need to mess around in traffic on Euston Road when the Underground would suffice. No madcap dash to hospital whilst in labour, the stuff of urban myth. No speed bumps, no shooting through the reds, no cold sweating taxi driver with an aggressive right foot and goosebumps all down his spine. (Or are those the marks from his seat-back beads making G-Force related imprints into his skin?)

Instead, we'd calmly got up, pulled on our clothes and walked collectedly down to the Tube station. We'd fed our tickets into the machine, sauntered to the platform and boarded the next westbound train as though we did this kind of thing every day. I'd wondered if someone would get up and offer me a seat. Or if I'd clear the carriage with the intrusion of my heavily pregnant, might-just-drop-it-now, cargo. As it happened, it had been half empty. We had shuffled in, sat down on a pair of adjacent seats and picked up a discarded copy of the *Metro*.

There was Mayor Ken with the Queen at his side, declaring City Hall open for business. Not sure what she found to smile about. The building, apparently, resembled a futuristic glass egg. One's son, for one, might have had a little something to say about HRH Mummy apparently throwing her (fuchsia-pink with coordinating floral bow) hat in with the monstrous carbuncles of London Towne.

I had folded the paper and tossed it back on the ledge behind me lest I should start to think I was back off to work, just another day. Same old, same old – today it was not.

It's been decided that I will have an elective caesarean.

The term elective caesarean seems to me to be rather a contradiction in terms. As though it's what I really *want* to do rather than what has effectively been decreed. Of course I *could*'ve gone ahead and insisted on giving birth to my breech baby naturally, but the midwives and medics all strongly advise the surgical route. I could still stamp my foot and go for it all gung-ho, give the midwives a bit of on-the-job variety and increase the number of vaginal breech deliveries in their portfolio to one. But I don't think I will. It'd be like asking a Kwik Fit employee to change a cranking handle. It may well be the case that you can't get better than a Kwik Fit fitter, but I wouldn't want to chance their vintage-motor handling skills, doing things in the 'old way', on me.

I'm not sure how I feel about it really. I don't like comparing myself to an old banger for starters. And I'm also scared of the idea of a C-Section, which makes a change from being scared of labour, I guess, but I'm not sure it helps.

In some ways I feel more than ever unexpectedly alone. No more safety-in-numbers bravado. No more security in the common bond I'd fostered with my labour-class contemporaries, joking companionably over the labour photo story we'd pieced together as a group, taking turns to clap a plastic dolly against our nervous chests, and gasping collectively at exhibit A, an epidural needle. Or exhibit 'eh?' as we preferred to call it. We'd been unequivocally together in this, even though then we barely knew each other's names. We were all from different backgrounds, with different accents, different values, different goals and different expectations. We'd only first met about six weeks previously, yet we were soon all bound in a sisterhood of labour-trepidation.

Except that I'm not in it anymore. I've swapped it for a private caesarean trepidation club instead.

The train had pulled into Euston Square. This was it then. Over the Top. Dirk had grabbed the bag that would surely now at last be dragged into full active service and I had stepped down onto the platform. Once through the barriers we'd taken a left and started to climb the stairs.

Lining the walls of the staircase was a fleet of ads for Gareth Gates's latest single, a 'Dial 999 for heart attacks' public awareness notice and a familiar glut of *Les Misérables* posters. I had briefly wondered what Victor would make of his literary baby having been so sold out. Might it induce in him a severe chest pain or perhaps he'd be well up for it and slavishly join in the hunt to sign up an angelic-voiced urchin to star in the role of Gavroche. Preferably one who could manage all the words in one go. (Sorry, Gareth, it's *chien* eat *chien* in Theatre Land, lovey.)

No sooner had we crested the top of the stairs, back within mobile coverage, than a familiar Nokia ringtone had tinkled, calling my husband to heel. Thinking that Dirk would let it go to voicemail, I'd continued out into the bustle of Euston Road and disappeared round the corner into Gower Street. And then I'd realised I was alone. He'd taken the call! Swooping back around the bend I'd found him in earnest conversation and looked askance at him over the receiver. He'd shaken his head meaningfully giving me a 'back off' glare. I'd glared back, wondering who he was talking to, the louse, before calling a truce, stepping back and watching the traffic stop-starting along Euston Road.

Once he'd rung off, Dirk had come apologetically back. 'Sorry, it just couldn't wait. Chris sends his regards.' His regards? Like, 'Happy major surgical operation!' 'Like, thanks!'

A few years later and I'm thinking of starting a new line of business: cards.

My children are invited to more parties than I am. (But that's not hard. I don't go to many parties. Certainly not to anyone's over the age of three.) To each one they must bring a present, a clean face and a card. I struggle. The clean face thing is really hard. We try making cards. We buy more than we make. There are, after all, only thirty-seven hours in the day.

It's not only for birthdays that cards are required. There are thank-yous and sorrys and missing-yous. There are good-lucks and congrats and welcome-to-your-new-homes. There are cards for mothers' days and fathers' days and you've-been-together-*how*-long days. There are cards, I'm reasonably sure, for step-mothers' days and godmothers' days and it's-all-blurring-into-one-big-haze days.

There are cards, I hear tell, for divorce congratulations. I'm not planning on receiving one but maybe I should hunt out a 'Blimey, we've been in the same country all week!' card? There are cards, and these I have had, for 12.5 year anniversaries. Or 12,5 *jaar*, to be precise. It's a big one in Holland, apparently. I think Hallmark UK's missing a trick.

I also got a 'Congratulations on Your Pregnancy' card from a colleague first time round. One to pop on the mantelpiece to ease the burden of spreading the news? One to slip conspicuously in your top pocket on the bus if you want to get a seat? One to remind you that you're *celebrating* when you're glumly staring another ginger biscuit and mug of elderflower tea in the face?

It kind of got me thinking. So many cards, yet so many missed opportunities. There's a whole raft of greetings cards out there just waiting to take their rightful place on the racks in Paperchase. What about:

• Cards for new dads-to-be: 'Congratulations, time to start drinking for two!'
• Good-luck-with-your-scan cards: includes complimentary

white pencil and integral blank black rectangle for the recipient to colour in at home.

- Our best wishes for the grandparents-to-be: a pop-up number with a spring-out mouth and a voice chip which, when card is opened, repeatedly says: 'In my day babies slept in the bottom drawer, swaddled and silent till they were at least sixteen and it never did you any harm, did it?' Footnote on the back cover of card reads: 'Irritating, isn't it? Even *you* shut it after a bit. Thanks in advance for refraining.'

- Happy Caesarean card: a deluxe little number with a 'Nil by mouth, don't give me cake!' badge, a complimentary tube of Nelson's arnica tablets and peppermint oil capsules for the wind sellotaped to the front. Text inside reads 'Have a sliced day!'

I wondered if I was beginning to hallucinate like a waif and stray in the desert. (Albeit a pretty hefty waif.) I'm nil by mouth but everywhere I look there's food. My swollen fingers are sausages. My puffy feet really do look like plates of meat, or at the very least a couple of sturdy pork pies.

This is it then. Time to face the heat. We arrive and walk up the couple of steps into the maternity hospital entrance. We nod to the security guard. He yawns. We go in and walk towards the lift.

I falter a little and gulp. It's been a long time in the making, but here we are at the door of our future. I feel a bit queer. Like those dreams you have when you're about to go into an exam but you realise you haven't read the set text.

I'm clutching Dirk's hand again as though to reassure myself he's still here. Still by my side, passport at home, mobile switched off. I know he's one hundred per cent there for me (well, one hundred per cent unless the noodles beckon). I know family and friends are rooting for us. I know that they know our programme and are thinking of us, probably even now. In spite of the reassurance of all that knowing, I'm suddenly struck by a tumbleweed moment. I'm in the heart of a thriving, noisy and smelly city, my husband by my side and the love and support of my nearest and dearest. But I can't help it, I still feel eerily on my tod.

I'm reminded of that small duffle-coated bear alone and far from home in the midst of a bustling London hub. He barely knew where he was, he'd no idea where he was about to go, but he coped with a hirsute stiff upper lip and a suitcase full of marmalade sandwiches.

Here am I, fresh off the boat from Darkest Highbury, and I feel as temporarily stranded as dear old Paddington. But things turned out OK for him and, pulling myself together, I tell myself I can follow in his Peruvian paw-prints. I may not be at liberty to comfort myself with marmalade sandwiches just now and I'm sure as heck I'm not as jauntily dressed as our hairy little friend (haven't come across any maternity duffle coats yet) but I'm ready to embark on my latest grand adventure with an open mind and a willing heart.

I briefly wonder if I should take a leaf from Michael Bond and name the young sprog after the place in which it arrives. But I figure if it's a boy then Elizabeth Garrett Anderson won't go down too well.

It's just the two of us. All calm and collected. We're buzzed in and walk to the labour ward reception desk. I'm on their list. Good start. I'm asked to take a seat in the waiting room. Less good. The walls of this unloved room would, I can see, soon start to grate. Having spent time in hospitals before I know that the cheery 'We'll call you through in a moment' could translate to anything between five minutes and five hours. I slump resignedly into an uncomfortable foam armchair while Dirk paces restlessly back and forth in a parody of the expectant dad itching to get down to the Jeremy Bentham. I absent-mindedly wonder if I should've packed a cigar with the Pot Noodle.

Before I've the chance to ponder Colombian or Costa Rican, however, we're staggeringly summoned to our next port of call. Stone me! And while I follow the midwife with go-faster stripes into the lift and up to level four it suddenly starts to feel more real than ever.

Upon our exit, we immediately find ourselves engulfed by dressing-gowned mums. There's one making a surreptitious call on her mobile in the stairwell, another clutching a packet of Marlboro Lights on her way down for a comforting fag. There's a drawn-looking woman in a wheelchair, pushed Benny Hill-style by a porter in pursuit of a nurse who's herself pushing a see-through fish tank on wheels. Out from the door labelled 'day room' comes another woman, clutching a slopping plastic jug of water. She briefly catches my eye and limps off, dragging a catheterised urine bag behind her. None of them look what you'd call glowing in the first bloom of motherhood. In fact, they all look a little sallow. Perhaps they're genuinely off colour or maybe it's just bounce-back off the vile yellow wall paint? Still, at least they're an effort at sunshine, which is more than can be said for the ward nurse who relieves Go-Faster Stripes.

Falling into step behind our unsmiling new chaperone, we're buzzed into the inner sanctum. I am now walking forth into the bosom of the post-natal ward, which feels rather odd given my immediate personal circumstances. I sense a reverential hush is required, as though I should be seen and not heard in the presence of my betters. I lower my head and walk meekly through the double doors when ... WHAM ... all thoughts of quiet are hurled out the window.

No sooner in than I'm knocked sideways by the noise of

animated chatter and whirring fans, the repeated ring of the demanding and largely unanswered ward phone, and the bleating cry of newborn babies. Babies! Here they are at last. I feel like Charlie walking wide-eyed into Wonka's factory and at last clapping eyes on a sea of chocolate. Here at last is a host of real babies. It is finally time to go and get mine.

Charm Offensive leads me to an empty bed and yanks the curtain ominously closed around us.

'You'll need to get into this ...' an inadequate-looking hospital gown is proffered in my direction '... and these,' a pair of above-the-knee compression stockings follow.

'Mmm. Even nicer than the woolly socks, then?' I venture nervously.

She looks poker-faced back at me and pulls a razor out of her pocket.

Gulp, it wasn't that bad a quip was it?

'You'll have to shave for the procedure. Would you prefer to do it yourself or shall I do it for you?'

'Sorry?'

'We need to shave the area for the incision before you go down to Theatre. I'll leave you to get changed and come back in five minutes' (five or fifty-five?) 'If you need me to do it, I'll shave you then.'

'Um, well, OK. Thanks.'

She slips out and half-draws the curtain again behind her. Dirk plonks the bag on the bed and sits down.

'So are you going to let Florence Nightingale have a go or is it going to be a DIY job?' he grins.

'Well, you know what they say: I would if I could but I can't.'

I look down at my protruding belly and can't imagine how I'd wield a razor blind and even dare hope to do anything but irreparable damage. I look at Dirk and my eyes narrow. Nope, he's an electric razor man by rule and I've seen the bloody nicks resultant of him trying out an occasional Gillette. On balance, I think I prefer Charm Offensive: the best a woman can get in the circumstances.

Some time later, and a little lighter off in the pubic hair department, I'm back in the lift descending to antenatal. I'd had my preparatory little chat and Q&A session with the anaesthetist and things seemed tickety-boo. But then someone realised they'd lost a sample of my bloods. They'd only taken out the odd gallon or so during the course of the pregnancy, but this particular one from the previous night's prepping session was apparently different (does blood change with time like a finely aged wine or a vinegary one if aerated for too long?) and today my veins are proving too tricky for Charm Offensive to get into. (Just my luck to have ended up with small veins in the genetic lottery of who gets what. 'So, this Charlotte then ... what'll it be? Small waist? Nah. Small thighs? Nah. Oh, I know, we'll give her those small veins we've had hanging around for a bit. Job done.')

And so, one or two unsuccessful jabs later (was Charm Offensive actually enjoying this?), it was decided I'd be better off seeing the phlebotomist, who is much versed in this kind of thing. What a job, I think to myself as I emerge from the lift amongst the fully clothed outpatients, self-conscious in my dressing gown and scanty hospital shift. And what an amazing job title.

Looking into my crystal ball, I wonder if I could've imagined the range of job titles I'd soon be able to claim as my own. I wonder if I'd have applied had I seen them on a card at the Job Centre.

Wanted - a combination of, or ideally all of the following:

- Rubbish Collector: needs to be constantly ready to accept sweet wrappers, banana skins and empty juice cartons. Only human dustbins need apply.
- Bag Lady: willingness to carry around crayons, spare age-2–3 undies and a large amount of plastic tat in handbag at all times vital.
- Show Girl: applicants must not expect showers or loo stops alone. Privacy doesn't come with this job.
- Entrepreneur: candidates should be able to think on feet. If you thought putting sellotape over your Sky card slot was a good idea, you're the right person for us.
- Mum: flexibility prerequisite as you'll automatically be answering to both your own and any other miscellaneous child that shouts out 'Mum' in public.

Actually, scrub all of the above. What's required is a Jackie O all trades. That's the female equivalent of an all-trading Jack. But if you can't manage glamour and the appropriate sunglasses, then a common or garden Superwoman will do.

Jobs and job titles. Sitting on the rubber-backed chair in the phlebotomist's tiny room and rolling up my sleeve, I feel incredibly remote from the world of work left behind not so very long ago. But then, am I? I am the client about to have as much blood sucked out of me as achievable in the shortest possible time. I'm due to pitch up at an important meeting soon, the exact timing of which is looking a little hazy due to heavy traffic. And I'd do well to keep my wits about me as I'm currently looking more than a little exposed from behind.

Thankfully, this time I'm able to deliver, obligingly squeezing out the requisite phials of blood after the phlebotomist trussed up my arm with a stretchy child's belt decorated rather curiously with Halloween motifs. A somewhat ghoulish accessory for one whose day revolves around extracting blood, I think. But no matter because it, ahem, does the trick.

This is no time to linger over corny Halloween gags, however, as a call to antenatal advises that a theatre slot's become free. It's all hands on deck. Or all hands rather imminently on me, you could say.

'Is it a boy?'

'No!'

'Is it a bat?'

'No!'

'Is it a boy-bat?

'No!'

'It's ... (tata ta tata ta tata ta drums) Bat Boy!'

'Yay!' (Crazy applause.) 'Super Bat Boy!'

Billy flounces round the living room fanning his polyester cape behind him, grinning dementedly through his dripping rubber fangs. He looks, quite terrifying. He's loving it.

Any excuse to plunder the dressing-up box. To shrug off our everyday clothes in favour of crazy hats, polyester trousers and Velcro belts.

Today Billy is Bat Boy. Sid's sporting a pirate hat. (Jack's at school in his uniform.) I am a princess. Naturally. I've had my face splodged with purple and black streaks. Billy was in charge of the face paints. The result is not exactly regal but the process was delicious. His face just inches from mine, breathing heavily in deep concentration, laden paintbrush whiskering nimbly over my nose and cheeks. By the end, I look like a hag. But I do, indeed, feel like a princess.

Before he is able to change his mind, Dirk is whisked off to scrub up and put on this season's must-have surgical outfit. As luck would have it, blue is his colour and I think he looks rather fetching. Not sure about the shower cap though. (Aren't they meant to go over your shoes?)

Time has now slowed. It's like a moving-through-water dream sequence. I look around and the room is suddenly filled with a motley cast of assembled extras. There's the butcher, the drugs-caretaker and the I-know-what-I'm-doing, just-let-me-have-a-try student faker. And someone else, another dropper-inner, a token VIP or two, me and Dirk and baby makes ten!

The *Muppet Show* theme tune crowds unwelcome into my head. I see Rowlf the Dog as the wisecracking Dr Bob with his lovely assistants Nurse Piggy and that blonde one with the eyelashes.

'Everything OK there, Mum?'

Everything's OK, I try telling myself. (Mum?) Everything's normal. Just another everyday procedure. Something they do all the time. Something I can smile through and handle just fine. After all, what's to get fussed about? I'm only about to have a crowd of people I've only just met whip off my last vestiges of modesty and delve into my exposed lower torso. No need to get my hypothetical knickers in a twist at all.

Whi ... stle, whi, whistle ... whistle. With a little whistle, whistle. Whi whi whistle, hmm.

'Here's a little song I wrote. You might want to sing it note for note.

'Don't worry.'

Clicky click, clicky click, clicky click.

'Be happy.'

Clicky click, clicky cl...

'Oh, Mummy,' groans Billy. 'Turn it off!'

'Why? I like it!'

'*I* don't. It's giving me a headache.'

Clicky click, clicky click, clicky STOP.

I turn it off. Shame. I was enjoying that. A bit of light-hearted retro fun on the radio station that never plays up-to-the-minute hits. The one all the painters and decorators listen to. They get a better result if they listen to, say, 'A Whiter Shade of Pale' or a bit of vintage Cream instead of that shocking Pink?

'Be happy,' I hum to myself in defiance of the ban.

'Stop singing!' boots in Billy, not one to let it drop while Jack, ever the mediator, suggests 'Can you put on the puddy cat one instead, Mummy? Please?'

'Peez,' adds Sid for his two penneth-worth.

'Oooh, *all right* then, suffering succotash!' I respond with my best Sylvester impression, which has them all, Billy included, in stitches.

Hello Children Everywhere: disc 3, track 6. PLAY.

I am a wittle tiny bird, my name is Tweety Pie
I wiv inside my birdcage, a hanging way up high...

To be fair, it's not my favourite. But then again, how can you deny them? They're all joining in with an approximation of the lyrics and/or madcap running around the kitchen in imitation (I think) of the bird. They're having fun. Ergo, I'm having fun.

It's all part of the game. I'm not worrying. And I am happy.

* * *

Before the Big Off an epidural is called for. This requires me to sit upright on the operating table. I lumber my bulk into the correct position and swing my legs over the edge, dangling them there like a small child. I'm entreated to take the pillow and curl myself around it in a ball. There's something very comforting about hugging something soft and fluffy.

'Soft and fluffy. Soft and fluffy,' I chant inwardly to myself. 'Soft and Lalala lala Land', fingers in ears, I am not listening to the muffled movements behind me. If I don't think about the large needle about to be jabbed into my spine then maybe it will go away.

Maybe it has? What are they up to? A series of fumbles, pauses, cold swabs and a bit more prodding takes place. 'Do we have a problem, Houston?' I eventually ask.

'Erm, no. The student anaesthetist's just learning the ropes and sometimes it takes a few goes.'

'Oh, OK then. You just take your time, I'm just hanging around. Nothing much better to do and all that...'

I'm on the point of trading in my 'soft and fluffy' chant for a rather louder but perhaps a little aggressive 'why are we waiting, we are suffocating ...' when all of a sudden BINGO!

The line is in, I'm lying down, they're under Starters' Orders. And they're off!

What would it look like, this game, anyway?

Official Mumopoly Game Rules

PLAYERS
This is a one-player game. The mummy may be aided or abetted by her other half, goaded or sloppy-kissed and/or

proposed to by her cast of children according to how the game progresses.

EQUIPMENT

The equipment consists of a broad game-plan board, two dice, lots of locks and plug covers, thirty-two baby vests and twelve extra drawers of baby-related gubbins. There are sixteen stair gates and sixteen nursing bras, twenty-four shape sorters (one for every hour of the day), and a large ugly fire screen.

The mummy is given $1,500. It is then all taken away from her. Better get it used to it, sucker. All remaining money and other equipment goes into the children's savings accounts. Go figure that one then.

BANKER

This – in some cases – is where the other half comes back in on the scene.

The banker may elect to conduct business close at hand – or arm's length – from all the action on the board.

It is his task to continue providing the $$$s to the mummy en route to their children. Whatever he does, he must not lose his job.

THE PLAY

The player selects a counter, or perhaps tries to juggle all six. There's a bootee, a Brio pull-along dog, a pirate ship, a cycling helmet and a Little Tikes car. Oh and something called an iron that some mums, well, this one at least, might not recognise any more. There are only so many hours after all ...

The player throws the dice to start. If you throw a

single, you can occasionally stop and have a cup of tea. If you throw doubles, you're really in trouble.

THE REST OF THE GAME
The rest of the game can pan out in one of many ways. Sometimes it can ... shh ... get a bit boring. The most important bits to look out for are:

- There are some squares with large question marks. There's one with a light bulb. Don't worry, it's the same for everyone. There are many more question-mark moments than light-bulb ones.
- There's a square called 'Free Parking'. Don't know about you, but there's no such thing as free parking round my way. Still, make the most of any offers of a free resting place. Especially if a cuppa and a biscuit are mooted.
- Try to avoid going to jail. That guy with the whistle looks like a grumpy park keeper reprimanding you or yours for walking on the grass. You can sit on 'Just Visiting' next to the ugly one behind bars if you're feeling ballsy. But take my advice. Don't mess with the Park Keeper.
- You will stumble into lots of dinky houses, all startlingly similar. None of them will be as messy as yours though. Don't sweat. Just try your best to make a run for it once awhile, preferably with the Banker.

END OF GAME
Oh no, that's right, I remember this game doesn't usually come with one of those.

Considering what they're actually doing it all takes a relatively short amount of time. I hadn't known how long it'd last or really what to expect of the knife-work itself. My cheery cousin Patricia, whose four-year-old bridesmaid I'd once been, had kindly taken it upon herself to call and talk me through her own caesarean experiences. She'd been gushingly reassuring and had likened the sensation to someone doing the washing-up in your tummy. This made it sound all cutesy and everyday acceptable and I'd liked her analogy at the time. But looking up today, the burly, masked surgeon standing squarely at my feet couldn't remind me less of a Fairy Liquid-toting Nanette Newman if he tried. And he's certainly not there to quickly rinse out the glassware; this man means serious pan-scrubbing business. 'Swab?' 'Check.' 'Scalpel?' 'Check.' 'Brillo pads?' 'Check ...'

I clap the oxygen mask closer onto my face and grip Dirk's hand a little tighter. I dip into a queasy patch, the anaesthetist notices and pumps in an antidote of some sort. I breathe a little easier and notice the strains of a radio somewhere in the background. Nelly is busy getting Hot in Herre. How appropriate I think as I lie here having managed, funnily enough, to take off nearly all my clothes.

I'm wondering why Nelly always seems to have a plaster on his face and what sort of a Band Aid I'll need for this when, sharp intake of breath, the moment is here. There's a hush and I'm suddenly numb. The fragile little form all bloody and vulnerable is pulled out of my stomach, up above the curtain for us both to see. I'm stunned. I don't even register the anticipated 'It's a boy/girl/baby!' cry at all.

I'm awash with emotions and hardly know my own name as they whisk off the baby out of range. The room is nothing but a blur. I turn my head to touch bases with Dirk. But he's not there. Oh blimey, he *has* keeled over after all I think with a flash of irritation.

But no, I'm in the wrong. Mr Squeamish, can't stand the sight of blood, ever, never, not on your clothed or unclothed Nelly has not only remained upright, he's also impulsively followed the paediatrician to the scales and Seen the Fright on the other side of the green curtain. Me, sliced apart, oozing blood; piece of cake. Two minutes into becoming a dad and he's already changing into a new man.

'He looks like his dad,' says the anaesthetist companionably, trying to make me feel included whilst the action's all happening elsewhere. Ah, a little boy then. Somehow this feels *right*.

Little Boy Blue, you've just been born.
Your mum's on cloud nine, your dad is airborne.
Where is the boy who makes our hearts leap?
'He's in Daddy's arms, fast asleep.'
'Will you wake him?'
'No, not I, For if I do, he'll be sure to cry because he wants feeding and I'm cacking myself about that bit.'

And now suddenly, here they are. Dirk approaches, eyes brimming with tears, a towel-wrapped bundle having been expertly placed in his arms. I feel myself welling up too and remind myself it is the baby who's meant to be crying. He'd had a fair go when they cleaned and weighed him but now seems to be dozing it off – plain stunned or just feeling more secure within his tight bindings, listening to his daddy's heartbeat.

Dirk hands my son across to me to hold for the first time. My chest is tight, my mouth is dry and I'm grinning from ear to ear. Top marks in terms of distraction techniques whilst my body's being sewn back together, though I'm not sure it'd work for all. 'Here, we've just got to suture up your appendix cavity, why don't you grab a hold of this convenient newborn to take your mind off things a bit?'

I look down into the face of my boy. He is tiny and red and all wrinkled up, there's blood still trapped in the folds of his skin and his eyebrows are a matted orange. Needless to say I know at once that he is perfectly beautiful.

Goodness only knows what had suggested to the anaesthetist that he looks like his dad though. Perhaps the pint-sized frown, perhaps the wrinkles or perhaps the eyebrows alluding to their shared Dutch genes and/or hair colour. Or maybe he just says that to all the girls. Because that's what we all want to hear. It's supposedly one of our natural instincts to immediately proclaim our newborn's resemblance to daddy as a sub-conscious means of convincing our partners that they really are the father.

The dads, meanwhile, are generally keen to point out the size of their sons' genitalia, those that have them. Sons, that is. I think we're fairly safe in saying that the dads have proven themselves perfectly adequately equipped in that department. I wonder how many times daily the tired midwives hear that 'chip off the old block' quip?

For myself, I can't really focus on whether he'll have Dirk's family jewels, my fingers or Grandpa's nose. All I care about is that he is, yup, a baby. Our baby. I can hardly take it in but as they say, seeing is believing. So I figure a spot of unashamed baby-gazing is the order of the day. Eyes down, here he is: one more man for the Moerman clan.

Dirk meanwhile is doing what blokes do best, fixating on numbers and charts. Our wee chap has apparently scored a perfect ten in his Apgar test. This – and I could see Dirk already envisaging Oxbridge – apparently means that he is top of the class in terms of heart and respiratory rates, muscle tone, reflexes and colour. I also think the fact he looks pretty good swaddled in white deserves a mention.

Whoever this Apgar was, he was obviously a man. Because before long my cuddle is interrupted by the need to perform another one of his tests on the little fella. Five minutes after the first. It's the done thing, it seems, to repeat all the rates and measures checks, just for luck. Apgar, Apgar, so good they perform it twice.

Whizzzz. Bang! Crackle crackle. Wheee!

I have a son. A small, blotchy-faced newborn son. He has a button nose generously sprinkled with tiny white pimples. He has a full head of fluffy baby-monkey hair, fair I see now the blood's all been washed out. And he is more breathtaking than an entire selection box of Deluxe Standard Fireworks. Hopefully not so noisy, though the jury's still out on that one at this stage of the game.

I look down into his crumpled face. He returns my gaze with uncomprehending, barely open eyes. He is an astonishingly calm little presence in the midst of a cacophony of life-changing firecrackers. I'm completely dizzy, meanwhile, as though I've just hitched a ride on a Catherine Wheel. What happens now?

Looking back with the benefit of hindsight, it comes to me in a flash. I did not need at that point Emma and her well-meaning but nauseating diary. I did not need the peppermint capsules (we were holding off on the bubbly. Trust me. Fizz and caesarean stomachs don't mix). And I did not need a CD with whale music, which is just as well really because I hadn't packed one.

What would've come in dead handy at the time, though, was a list of clear, bulleted instruction on how to handle my bursting little box of colourful starbursts, twilight glitters and whistling crackle mines.

Here, perhaps, is how it would've looked:

- Only accept a baby that complies with BS 8487
- You should be aware that it is intended for Indoor, Garden *and* Display use: 'Ooh, that's a fresh one. Let's have a closer look at you then, coo-che coo-che coo coo'
- Keep babies in a sealed pram or Moses basket until you're good and ready to handle them
- Follow the baby's instructions carefully: Cry = hungry. Cry = wet. Cry = wind. Cry = tired (C'mon now, keep up)
- Use a torch or hand lamp if you're feeling in the dark. Never use a naked flame
- Cuddle one at a time (hug-hungry adults *must* learn to share) and wear gloves
- Wind at arm's length using a suitable muslin. Observers should stand well back
- Ensure all well-meaning but frequently explosive older children are well supervised
- Keep all pets and animals behind closed doors
- Never put babies in your pocket
- Never throw babies

Despite annual safety warnings, the first week of a new baby still ends in hormonal tears for far too many utterly kiboshed new mummies.

Babies can provide fun and entertainment, but only if everyone follows the right safety procedures and remembers provoking a stressed new mummy is like a red rag to a bull. Hormones can be very dangerous if misused.

Remember; only dial 999 in an emergency.

Like all good shortlists, we'd spent hours agonising over it. We'd chosen random daft names from the Baby Names book, proposing suggestions with studiously straight faces, daring one to question the other's bluff. We'd strung schoolboy-snigger combos together for a Beano-style laugh ('How about Brian Uranus Moerman?'). And we'd done that thing where you close your eyes, flick the pages and arbitrarily stick a needle in. 'And the choice of the needle today is ... Mitch!' 'Hmm, if at first you don't succeed, eh?'

The due date came closer; we decided to pull ourselves together. We drew up a favourites list that'd help us to focus but still leave our options open. We had a list of top five for boys and top five for girls. And then we'd disregarded it entirely.

I know. Let's call him Jack. And so Jack he will be.

By the time we're back on the ward, he's been named and announced to the family by text. Though the message is timeworn – 'Jack Moerman, 6lb 3.5 oz, Mother and Baby doing fine' – the means of conveying it is a thoroughly modern one.

And now we're attempting to get comfy in the sweltering fourth-floor Nixon Ward. Why is it always so warm in hospitals? The yellow curtain hangs hot around my bed. I'm utterly immobile. Dirk sits tucked in beside me on another tired foam armchair. Baby Jack lies asleep, feet to the foot of a cot in which he looks lost. He is enveloped in a battle-worn NHS cellular blanket because newborn babies *must* be properly wrapped up just in case the ward temperature should suddenly plummet from tropical to Arctic when no one's paying attention.

Jack is kept company by a blue cardboard teddy bear displaying all his credentials.

Baby's name: Baby Moerman (non-imaginative parents, then)

Baby's number: 68217864 (prolific parents, then?)

Mother's name: Mummy (dhurr)

Date: 24/7 (aka the non-flexible hours that come with the job)

Time: 10.56 a.m. (just in time for elevensies!)

Weight: 6 lb 3.5 oz. Or 2.822 kg (Means nothing to me. I count in Old Money, don't you?)

Type of delivery: Caesarian Section (You'd think they could spell it right by now?)

Head circumference: 32 cm (bursting with brains eh ... what's average anyway?)

Length: 50 cm (his body length, Daddy, his *body* length)

We sit, we admire, we lose ourselves in the wonder of admiring his tiny fingers and toes, the remnants of soft lanugo hair and the angry purple birthmark behind his ear. Everybody's babies are, of course, perfect. It's just that ours is *more* perfect.

My parents come to visit. We are showered with hugs, gasps of wonder and a barrelful of hearty pats on the back. Well, except for me, I'm still lying immobilised on mine. Flowers and fruit arrive. And a nurse to clean me up since, unbeknownst to me, I've been slowly seeping blood into the sheets.

I suddenly see what it will be like to be old.

Chapter 8

The car draws slowly up, stops, sweeps fluidly backwards and in. Ah, the beauty of a perfectly executed parallel park. Maybe one day, I'll be able to do it too. Dirk turns off the ignition and pulls on the handbrake. I peel myself off the back seat where I've been hovering agitatedly over Jack this last hour or so.

'A few days old and he's already treating you like a taxi driver,' I'd quipped as the car inched along in rush-hour traffic, the sun beating down, unforgiving on our hot tin box. Our home-grown cabbie didn't see the humorous side.

My cotton T-shirt's sticking damply to my back. Dirk leans in from the open door on the other side. Our heads meet in the middle and we fumble inexpertly together over the car seat clip. 'WARNING' says the bright yellow label inches from our faces. 'DANGER OF DEATH!' That's cheerful, I think. Makes a change from the usual nursery decorative bunnies or those bizarre pastel hippos.

Luckily Jack doesn't look in any imminent danger of being biffed by an air bag or a large sub-Saharan African mammal that I can see. But I'm aware there are hidden dangers lurking around every corner. I should know: I've just broken a nail trying to unclick this adult-proof car seat.

'Here. Let me see.'

Click-Clunk! Well thank heavens for that. It's the inverse sound effect of the road safety campaigns of yore but no less satisfying. Dirk grabs the arched handle and waits for me as I clamber inelegantly out of the car. We grab hands and walk gawkishly up the garden path together. Hi honey, we're home!

Our home is more or less the same as all the other houses up and down the street. The Bovis homes of their time. All the same and all built in neat rows. We have the same privet hedge as a hundred others up and down the neighbourhood, the same iron coal-chute cover just before the front door, and the same worn old flagstone slabs that have welcomed men, women, children and Health Visitors into the house for decades.

(Sorry, I don't remember inviting you? 'Come in then,' through gritted teeth and witness at first hand the grubby baby mewling at my breast, yesterday's breakfast bowls still in the sink, my hair unwashed since the beginning of time. 'Yes, I'm coping just fine, thanks!')

But of course, the house isn't completely identikit. The march of time has added variation and character to the bricks and mortar just as much as to the occupants. The finial above our front door is missing. We've a green but non-flowering Wisteria scrambling up the front wall. And our privet hedge has an air of smug self-satisfaction about it. For this is no ordinary hedge. It is the hedge, no less, that Colin Firth stroked in the closing scenes of *Fever Pitch*. Well, OK, so maybe it was the bush next door if you're being finicky. But you're not telling me Colin didn't stroke ours in rehearsal?

This is the house in which Jack spilt his milk.

This is the hand
That held the mug

That fell in the house in which Jack spilt his milk.
This is the Billy
That jogged the hand
That held the mug
That fell in the house in which Jack spilt his milk.

This is the Sid
That bit the Billy
That jogged the hand
That held the mug
That fell in the house in which Jack spilt his milk.

This is the mummy all forlorn
That despaired of the Sid
That bit the Billy
That jogged the hand
That held the mug
That fell in the house in which Jack spilt his milk.

This is the friend with a teapot warm
That made the tea for the mummy all forlorn
That despaired of Sid
That bit the Billy
That jogged the hand
That held the mug
That fell in the house in which Jack spilt his milk.

This is the house to which I will bring my babies home. This is the house in which I'll sit and drink endless cups of tea, discussing hopes, fears and screams with my dear friend Avril and others.

Dirk unlocks the door and steps in first with his lopsided load. I hobble over the threshold behind him. Carrying the car seat without a) doing yourself a mischief, b) looking like a resident of Notre-Dame or c) providing white-knuckle entertainment for the jostled-about occupant within looks a whole new art to learn. Must've missed that bit in the NCT classes. Still, I've got about six weeks to watch, learn and snigger before I'm allowed to lift heavy loads.

The method appears to be as follows:

- Stand with upper torso at an angle of approximately 25 degrees
- Use offside arm (lower shoulder) to stabilise, stretching it out at approximately 45 degrees, palm down and fingers extended groundwards
- Hunch nearside shoulder upwards, pointing elbow towards the wall. Suspend infant seat from nearside lower arm and Bob's your back-injury clinic patient

'What's funny?'

'Ooh. Nothing. You just look like you're about to lift him up and pour him out that's all.'

'What?'

To say I'm relieved to be home is an understatement. I'm ecstatic. I feel I've just picked up my Get out of Jail Free card – a jail that was forever hot, smelling of other people's food, and with baths that I literally wouldn't set foot in – and I'm loving it. OK, so I'm a tad uncomfortable with my niggling war wound. But look, here are a stash of cards and presents to open as though it's my birthday. There'll be my own mug that I can drink a decent cuppa from. There'll be my kind of food to eat, a *comfortable* chair to sit in and my own bed in which to sleep, albeit interruptedly. I feel like one of the three bears returning home from my wanderings. Let's hope Goldilocks didn't pick the locks and sabotage it all while I was out.

Dirk plonks the car seat down in the middle of the living room. It looks a bit small and lost. I note the absence of empty porridge bowls and broken chairs and heave a sigh of relief. Looks like we're alone, then. Just the way we want it.

We've ring-fenced the first few days as time to ourselves before the family descends. I've heard all that stuff about not working with children and animals and seen the black-and-white clip of the elephant pooing on John Noakes at least twice. So I'm not going to let our newborn in sheep's clothing get one up on us in front an audience. Not until we've had a few days' grace to acclimatise to our wriggly unpredictable little blind date and him to us that is.

He's twitching noiselessly in the carrier. His intense blue eyes are open and trying to focus on something just above his head. It may be the arched handle which until a moment ago was clasped by Daddy's strong pink fist, it may be the dust particles in the air which are strangely new and exciting when you've been cooped up in a womb for nine months, or it may be the imaginary think bubble floating in the air above him: ... o o O O O ('So what happens next then?'). Good question, son. I see he's got an enquiring mind. Chip off the old block. So, erm, what does happen next?

. . .

Abracadabra
Bambi the deer
Make the old Charlotte
Disappear!

Whoosh!

Wow. Now that's what I call magic.

I'm sitting on the sofa with all the stage props. I've a muslin cape swathed around my shoulders, a sparkly teaspoon which I'm swirling confidently round and round, and a large book of tricks that rests within arm's reach at all times. To be fair, there's still a large L sign hanging from my back. I don't yet know *all* the tricks (transforming screaming banshee into docile lamb anyone?) but my plan is to swot up and join the Magic Circle asap. ('Oh, please!' she says, remembering the all-important magic word.)

Doo dooby doo dooby doo dooby doo doo. Doo dooby doo dooby doo dooby doo doo.

(This is organ filler music in case you're wondering when Shaggy and Scoob are going to wonder in on set, or indeed start to envisage me up to my elbows in the doo doo which does, I grant you, frequently happen but not in this particular scene.)

'Ladies and gentleman, boys and girls, let's hear it for the one, the only, the Great Mummy Marveloso!'

(Applause)

> Abracadabra
> Rumbling tummy
> Make this Charlotte
> Into a mummy!

> Whoosh!

I drink Rooibos tea. I instinctively rock supermarket trolleys whether or not there's a small person inside. And there's a large swathe of people who don't know my Christian name at all, for now I have become 'Jack's mum'.

Ooh. That's good.

Abracadabra
Twitchety mouse
Bring a baby
Into this house!
Whoosh!

Half the contents of the house leaps up onto a high shelf. The laundry basket begins to mushroom. A nappy disposal bin materialises in the bathroom, looking like a pint-sized lemon Dalek, smelling like something far more evil. The bath steels itself for being pooed in. I'll chuckle about it (possibly) until the time that I'm sharing the tub.

The bath is the epicentre of change in our house. A bath alone? Ah yes, I remember those. Vaguely. Bath times are now a veritable jamboree. Declare it's time for the bath and it is as though someone's fired a starting gun. Bang! And they're off! They strip, they squeal and they would happily carouse around the house playing hysterical pre-bath games nude till the cows come home.

As we don't generally expect a herd of Friesians to come wandering in, I eventually have to call time, grab the three white-bottomed absconders and plonk them in the bath. And that's when the real fun and games begin.

If they stay in the bath that is. Fairly often Jack does his best 'In the Box' impression by jumping out of it. The bath, that is. Needing to answer the call of nature usually. Billy invariably runs off just while I'm putting Sid in and if he escapes all mayhem breaks loose. He'll be off, skipping around the hallway, daring me delightedly to come and get him. I don't. I will not leave the other boys unattended. Apart from the time Billy bellowed 'Mummy, there's a *man* in the loo!' which got me running super quick. Luckily it was just a Playmobil man that Sid had dropped in earlier. (Though arguably not so lucky for *him*.) I heaved a sigh of relief, held the 999 call and hauled my slippery fish of a son into the bath with the others. Just another nice relaxing bath time ...

Once I have them all in, they clamber unselfconsciously about, happily ensconced together in the Matey bubbles. Occasionally tweaking willies ... not always their own. There's a glut of ubiquitous plastic toys, sodden flannels (often airborne), a series of excitable shrieks and an unrelenting splash fest. When they've finished their evening's ablutions, the floor invariably ends up looking like post-event Glastonbury.

But for all their crazy-nut and room-soaking bathtime antics, it's still one of my favourite magic moments; seeing all three of my blond-haired cherubs lined up in a row, all naked. Horsing around with bubble-bath beards, giggling at the dot-to-dot nobbly bath-mat imprints on everyone's bums, squealing at the sighting of the small and forebodingly dark toy submarine, mistaken by all for a Sid-related accident.

Rub-a-dub-dub, mayhem in a tub.

Fun times.

'Shall we get him out then?'

'Yes, let's.'

I sit gingerly down on the sofa, mindful of my healing wound. Dirk brings the baby seat within my reach, lets me manage the straps even though I can't yet lift the child. There's a fresh bout of fumbling while I wrestle with the next confounding clip. I feel a twit, awkwardly incapable once again. My son is watching me with quizzical eyes. Of all the car seats in all the towns in all the world, she had to walk into mine.

'What's the problem?' asks Dirk. 'Got two left thumbs?'

Don't you just hate it when they say things like that?

'I'm trying my best. It's just that it requires a knack. Which I don't yet have.'

Ah, there we go. Released. I got there in the end, eh? Dirk squats, inches his hands in under the warm white bundle that is our newborn son and lifts him onto my lap. He is as light as a feather. Here's looking at you, kid.

'How does that feel, then?'

'Erm. Terrifying, to be honest.'

'Why?'

He seems so small and fragile and I'm worried I might break him. What an enormous, gut-wrenching responsibility to have and to hold in my clumsy, novice arms.

'It just feels so huge.'

'But he's tiny?'

'No. Yes, I know, but I mean "it". Everything's changed. All for him. This tiny wee mite whose neck could snap if you don't hold him right.'

'Oh surely, he's more robust than you think.' Dirk sits next to me and threads his arm comfortingly round my shoulder. 'You'll soon get used to it.'

But it's not just about the here and now, and holding his matchstick neck up right. It's about life as we know it from now on in.

'It'll be OK. It's what you wanted. What we wanted.'

'Yeah, I know, but I'm still feeling scared.'

I'm feeling small on the threshold of something big. Everything I've known up until now has been junked into the big black bin liner with my defunct files, my business cards and the packet of past-its-sell-by-date Slim-a-Soup. What's left is a swirling vat of expectations. All of them centring on the tiny guy who's currently nuzzling into my T-shirt. Will I handle him right today? Will I handle him right in five, ten, twenty years' time? Will I go the distance and be a good mum to him till death us do part? How will I know what to do? Or if what I've done is OK?

I sigh and look down into his blotchy red face. My heart performs a reflex lurch. OK, so there are no flat-pack assembly instructions, no KPIs or targets, not even a 'this way up' arrow, but I'm going to damn well try my hardest on this one.

Just think of the car seat, I resolutely decide. If at first you don't succeed, just bumble along till something clicks and surely you'll get there in the end.

It is now early evening. The sun's still hot and high and we're reclining in deckchairs. Behind us looms the Arsenal away fans' stand which abuts the garden. Our shorts-topped legs stretch languorously towards the house. This is the life. Can't understand what all the fuss is about. Jack's sleeping like a ... well, sleepy baby and we're just taking it easy for a bit.

So this is the Brick Wall Dad was always going on about? Don't really get it. I chuckle briefly to myself recollecting the doodles we used to scrawl across our pencil cases in school. There was this beady-eyed bald bloke who'd peer with his nose hooked forward over the top of a brick wall.

'Wot no trauma-rama?' I allow myself to think a little smugly and consider making a cup of tea. If I can rouse myself to switch on the kettle. Which I decide I can't. But then I take an anxious look at my watch. How long since Jack has last fed? How long has he now been asleep? Is it normal? Is he OK? I jump up with a start to go and check up on him. Still snoozing peacefully.

Seconds behind me, Dirk comes into the kitchen hot on my fidgety heels. 'Everything OK?'

'Erm, I think so. Just not sure if I should wake him up for another feed.'

'Er. Dunno.' Pauses. 'How long's it been?'

'Two hours, seventeen minutes.'

'Oh.'

'Do you think he's still OK?'

'Er. Dunno.'

We both lean ponderously over the basket and wonder together in silence.

I feel like I'm in one of those dreams when you know you should be somewhere, but you don't know where and there's no way of finding out. You think you should be in double maths, but you can't remember where you wrote down your timetable and you're too ashamed to ask because you *ought* to know and in any case, you wouldn't be sure who to ask. Have you missed something, will you be found out?

'Wot, no timetable?' the bald-headed wall-gazer is now gloating meanly at me. Day one back at home and I haven't yet shoe-horned my baby into a routine. Will it all go terribly wrong from here on in? I reach for the neglected copy of Gina Ford's paperback, which hasn't been opened since I wrote my 'how many vests' shopping list.

The androgynous naked baby floating through the clouds on a huge red feather gazes confidently back at me. 'The secret to calm and confident parenting' the cover proclaims. 'This book could be your salvation!' Great, just what the doctor ordered, I'd thought when I bought it.

And indeed it had been a great help when I'd dithered over the prerequisite number of vests and socks and shawls. It had pointed me helpfully towards black-out curtains, a baby monitor and even some of this Napisan stuff that I'd not, until that moment, had the pleasure of being introduced to. I'd gaped reverentially over the laundry advice, skimmed distastefully past the nipple-cream pages and then tossed the book to one side in favour of the baby names ones which were, let's face it, far more interesting at that point.

But now I'm wondering whether I should've been more assiduous in my preparing-for-baby homework. Should I have carved out a timetable and slapped it decisively onto the fridge? Should I have already been acclimatising myself to breakfast 'no later than 8 a.m.' in lieu of making the most of my soon-to-be-extinct lie-ins? Should I have sourced purveyors of outsize crimson feathers just in case I missed the bit where they became absolutely vital?

Frantically, I thumb at lightning speed through the couple of hundred odd pages and wonder if I can cram it all in before Jack surfaces. He simply isn't going to swallow the excuse that my carefully planned routine has been eaten by the dog. (We don't have a dog.)

And so skipping the shopping instructions (well there's a first for everything) I flick to the pages on establishing a routine. Ah, here's the kind of thing I need. Only it's not. From my quick-skim approach to digesting a whole ream of facts, figures, timings and commands, I soon deduce that everything's worked out for babies who weigh seven pounds or above. Well that's put the kibosh on that one then.

In any case my 6 lb 3.5 oz baby is now bleating for attention so sod the book and sod the routine. This tiny guy is making it abundantly clear that he needs feeding NOW!

Jack does not eat mushrooms.

I once tried to slip some on top of a pizza, hiding them under the cheese, but he rumbled me. He *never* eats mushrooms. Billy does not eat scrambled eggs. Or noodles. Or cauliflower. And he's not too keen on rice. Sid does not eat pasta.

When I'm considering what to feed them, I often wonder if I

should make a pie chart. Not a fish pie one, obviously, it'd only get poo-pooed. I worked out yonks ago that fish pies will never work on the basis of the rule of thumb that the longer a meal takes to prepare, the less they're likely to eat it.

No, I feel it would be handy to draw up one of those three-circled pie charts and bung it on the fridge. If a + b like beef but c prefers chicken, what on earth, peering into the almost empty fridge, shall Mummy cook for tea?

What do we reckon? Oh, of course. Looks like it might have to be Heinz Baked Beanz? (I could cosh that Z with a wooden spoon, couldn't you?) It's one of the holy grail items that lurk in the gothic triangle in the middle of the pie, a subset of all three's approved lists. Just to create a full picture, cabbage, red peppers and tinned fruit all float about in the ether, resolutely in the category of things that no one will touch with a barge pole.

It is more complex than advanced maths, feeding three small children. I struggle even with basic maths. If 1 mother + 3 small children each with different tastes and rates of hunger = lots of head scratching + baked beans on toast, then feeding one small baby who is unable yet to demand crisps, chocolate eggs and cheese strings = easy peasy, surely.

Right? Wrong.

It is 2 a.m. It's hot and sticky. Jack is crying agonisingly. So will I be, soon. I'm trying to get him to latch on but it's just not working right like it did in the hospital. He's clearly famished, but the milk bar appears to be closed.

They've all hammered on about flesh-to-flesh being helpful, though this is clearly misguided. 'You can't be serious,' I'd wanted to point out, 'he's British, I'm British. We don't *do* unnecessary skin-to-skin contact. Or even fully clothed contact for that matter.' But now it's the middle of the night and everyone's desperate, I'm prepared to overlook etiquette. I'd even jump a queue if I saw one.

The theory is I'm like his own personalised Air Wick FreshMatic. I've been the one fragrancing his warm and comfortable living room for the last nine-odd months, therefore the best way to calm him down and make him feel all snug and happy with the world again is to give him a quick spritz of *eau de moi*, which means getting up close and personal with not a lot on. Only my essential oils canister thingummy must've run out. Either that or my 'outside smell' is just too different from my 'inside smell'. Must be all the sweat and sniffled tears I'm exuding. (No blood as yet, though the way this child's been chewing on my nipples, 'tis but a matter of time.)

It's our first night back from the hospital. Even though Jack slept calmly all afternoon, he seems to have risen again like a horror-flick banshee now that night has fallen. My baby is angry. He's helpless. He's clearly downright starving.

'Can't you try the other side?' suggests Dirk helpfully.

'I've *tried* the other side.' I respond through gritted teeth. 'He's just not ...' I manage to jam his mouth onto my nipple and he gnaws ravenously for a brief magic instant. To no avail. Within seconds he's back off again, mouth wide and screaming, face a furious crimson.

'Well we've got to do something,' Dirk says, sitting upright now. 'This clearly isn't right.'

'I know it's not right.' I must be doing something wrong. I just don't know what. I just don't know what to do next.

The LED clock taunts 2:13, the central dots flashing me mockingly. I feel hollow and helpless, stuck in the middle myself. I know I need to take control of the situation, stick the flag in the ground and assert myself as a mother. This is the first night of the rest of our lives. I need to respond now as I mean to go on. So I open the floodgates and start to cry full tilt.

The result is a wicked snowball effect. The more upset I get the more frantic Jack seems to be. The more distraught he is, the more the back-seat driving seems to grate. If I don't do something soon, I'm going to roll out of control to the bottom of the hill and go SPLAT on a picket fence.

I call the midwives in a state of delirious panic. The ward phone rings for an eternity and then a terse voice picks up. I gabble a few words about our panicky plight, about my fears for the baby's well-being. I don't mention my fears for my own sanity or the imminent black eye that Dirk's severely in danger of incurring.

'Can't it wait till morning? We're very busy.'

'Well, it's just ...' I snivel, trying to grasp out at the fast-slipping-away lifebelt.

We'd been packed off home with our discharge files and some numbers to call in case of difficulty. At a loss for how to stop the hysterical crying, Dirk had whisked the red-faced bundle off my chest and insisted I ring for help. I'd called the first number hoping for what, a matey AA man to roar up, prop up a warning triangle and sort us all out very nicely thank you very much?

Clearly the ward nurse, who'd encouraged us to ring and just AAsk if we'd the slightest worry, hadn't genuinely meant to offer herself as the fourth emergency service. I realise now we'd been mere house guests who'd outstayed our welcome, waved off with an insincere 'Let's not leave it too long next time, see you again soon (but not *too* soon, I jolly well hope)' send-off.

I ring off, glance at Dirk pacing up and down with the squalling baby and gulp back a fresh barrage of tears. Next on the list is the community midwives' number. If at first you don't succeed blunder tearfully on, I think, as I tap the numbers into the keypad.

'Well, he's new to the game just like you,' says the not overly sympathetic voice at the end of the line. 'You're both beginners. Sometimes it just takes a while. Why don't you try to express some and see if he'll take it from the bottle? Or you could give him some formula just to tide him by?'

'But I ...' the phantom voice thief steals up behind and grabs me. I whimper numbly down the phone.

'Lots of mums find it hard at first. And if you've had a C-Section, maybe the milk's just not come in yet. Really, you shouldn't worry. If you're still having problems in the morning, you could go and see your Health Visitor for help.'

As the moon peeks through the curtain at our dishevelled bed and the flurry of distraught activity inside our bedroom, the morning seems an awfully long way off.

It's raining, it's pouring,
The babe at last is snoring.
I lost my head
My nips are in shreds
I'll be totally knackered by morning.

It's now nearing nine. Gina has decreed that I need to be up, dressed and breakfasted before eight. I briefly think I'd like to push Gina's face into a bowl of freshly poured Crunchy Nut corn flakes. But that'd be unkind. In this day and age. Maybe just the plain corn flakes without the nuts would do the job. You can never be too careful.

It's the morning after the night before. I'm absolutely bushed. It's been a hellish twelve hours. After lots of huffing and puffing, weeping and not much sleeping, we'd eventually crashed in a bundle of exhaustion around dawn. Sleep is the cure of all evils. Or just a welcome release from the diabolical dream sequence that actually turned out to be reality.

Had she really said it or had I been hallucinating? Did we genuinely think that the idea of having a maiden bash at expressing milk in the dead of night might be in any way shape or form helpful? Me with my milk 'not yet come in' had torn off the cling film from the breast-pump box like a woman possessed. I'd previously handled it with a mixture of mild horror and disgust. Now I looked on it as the answer to my prayers, a nugget of gold, glinting in the sieve after an eternity of desperate panning. Fool's gold, as it turned out.

Dirk jiggled the fretful baby and tried to read the instructions. I poured myself into the funnel, stood upright again and squeezed the handle. In the broad light of day, it seemed comical (possibly). In the dim pre-dawn light it had not.

And then what was this bit about ... shh ... formula? I'd spent the previous several months visiting antenatal clinics whose walls were adorned with pictures of rosy teenage mums, knowing-looking dads and poleaxed begetters of twins all proclaiming that Breast is Best. We'd had it drummed into us until we stood in glazed lines with dull eyes, gently nodding heads and gaping mouths repeating a 'we will breastfeed, we will breastfeed, we will breastfeed' mantra as though there was no tomorrow.

But now, at the first hurdle some midwife at the end of the phone in the middle of the night had breezily suggested I 'just top up with a little formula to tide him by'. It was like a red rag to a bull. By jiminy, I'd resolved, I am not going to be tempted to eat of the apple that quickly, my dear friend. Oh no. By hook or by crook, I *will* breastfeed this child. Even if my nipples start to look and feel like that red rag *after* the bull's finished with it.

* * *

It is Monday. We've had the whole weekend to get used to parenthood. We're now seasoned pros. The number of nappies I've changed has moved into double figures. I've worn the vomit-on-shoulder badge of honour at least twice. And the bags under my eyes have already moved in, plonked themselves down and look set to stay for the duration. It's a future vision of terminal five and it's not a pretty sight.

I also *think* that my milk has finally come in. I'm not bursting like a Friesian at milking time. But I seem to be able to silence and satisfy my little boy by letting him nibble to his heart's content while I veg in front of the TV. I'd never before devoted any more than five minutes to watching *Ground Force*. They'd said parenthood would change you, but I never thought it would involve spending inordinate amounts of time in the company of Alan Titchmarsh. With my top off.

All of this, needless to say, has been going on behind closed doors. I've never been an exhibitionist, so frankly my exposed torso can remain for Alan's eyes only. This being the case, I feed with the curtains firmly closed, day or night. They say my jaundiced baby needs sunlight, but they must be having a laugh if they think I'm going to sit outside half-dressed next to a football stadium. It may be out of season, but I know for a fact they've a large replay screen for selected highlights and I'm not prepared to risk it.

The closed doors behind which I am generally lurking are to be found in the following delightful four-bedroomed property:

Four-bedroom house, Highbury, N5
About the property (Ref: TILII)
Presented to a mediocre standard, this bog-standard four-bedroomed Victorian house enjoys a smattering of original, replica and sadly busted period features set

within average-sized rooms over a higgedly-piggedly arrangement of floors.

The property comprises:

- Double reception room complete with the usual stacks of cushions, a couple of restful woodland-walk paintings and a soporific ticking clock. The colour scheme is predominantly blue. Perhaps the owner is in need of calming and/or has a soft spot for Duncan James.

- Kitchen, Shaker-style. Shaky crayon drawings on wall behind curtain pending. Language used when negotiating newly fitted cupboard locks not generally Shaker-approved.

- Cellar. Full of crap. Plus large bus wheel left by previous occupants. Drunken student prank perhaps? Harder to dispose of in cold light of day than orange flashing light. Far better to leave for future under-five occupants to gape and marvel at. 'It's a REAL bus wheel! Wow!'

- Four bedrooms, one of which is now 'the nursery'. Best-fitted-out room in house. Furnishings include cot, musical mobile, digital baby monitor, plug-in night light, room thermometer, blackout blind, dimmer switch, obligatory A.A. Milne prints, flock of cuddly toys and, last but not least, a height chart for stoking 'my one's bigger than yours' inter-parent competition.

- Bathroom with battleship-grey fittings that ran aground sometime in the seventies. Upgrade planned. Having bath alone also planned by owner, sometime later this month, if lucky.

- Long, thin and average garden to the rear overlooked by distinctly non-average neighbour, Highbury Stadium. The garden boasts close proximity to the away fans' stand and as such affords the owner rich and varied language lessons, specialising in expressions that point out the ineptitude of one's hosts. (Present owner hopes presents owner's new son isn't paying too much heed.)

The house is situated on a litter-bin-lined residential street, some of which are used on match days. The exclusive range of shops, cafés and dry cleaners of Highbury Barn are also close by. Travel links Arsenal Underground Station (Piccadilly Line) and Finsbury Park Station (British Rail, Piccadilly and Victoria lines) or the number 19 bus. Still a Routemaster at the time of writing, but don't hang about if you fancy a ride.

Total Sq Ft: quite a few (approx), most of which will soon be littered with a glut of plastic tat, seasonal leaf collections and a flood of unsolicited toy and children's clothes catalogues.

Dirk's clearly a bit put out by my sudden allegiance to Alan. He's stopped suggesting which breast I use next. He's laid off trying out nocturnal breastfeeding as a spectator sport, preferring (sheesh) to carry on sleeping. And he's mysteriously taken to disappearing randomly out into the garden while I fuss over the Moses basket inside. You can wink, Dirk, but you'll never lay out a bed like Titchmarsh I say ...

I soon work out he's not dead-heading the roses though or testing his Yorkshire accent out of earshot of the house. Disappearing into the shed on the pretext of grabbing his rake is just a front to cover his dirty secret. He's back on the mobile phone. And he's plotting.

'Erm, Charlotte?'

'In the living room. Feeding again!'

He ambles cautiously through.

'Everything OK?'

'Yeah, he's quiet now. Must've been hungry again.' I don't know very much about babies yet. But what I do know is that if I latch him on, he stays quiet, I can sit down for a while and if my brain's not gone on all-out strike I can start piecing together where I last left the remote control.

'Look, I'm sorry to do this to you. But the thing is, there's this client meeting. It's really important that I go.'

I gaze blankly at him.

'It's Chris. He says it'll only be an hour or two. I'll be back before you've noticed.'

I narrow my eyes, shift back a little into the cushions and my blank expression morphs into animation.

'What? What is it?'

'It's fine. I've just realised I'm sitting on it.' I say cheerfully.

It is Tuesday afternoon. I'm in the kitchen, alone with my son for the very first time. Result! If I want to I can turn on some cheesy music, crank it up loud and measure up the mettle of my boy. Are you, son, hereby more of a Sinatra or an Elvis kind of guy?

I decide on balance to leave off 'Jailhouse Rock', savouring the silence instead. It's eerily quiet. Jack's fast asleep, his fists bunched up tight beside his head. His arms form a perfect strong-man pose, the top of an H shaped rugby post. He's not, of course, very strong at all. Neither am I.

The room is filled with the heady scent of the deep-purple lilies that Dirk's client Chris has sent in apology for spiriting him off. I've never before received such luxurious flowers. They're tall and stately and as dark as night. The colour of bruises.

The curtains are pulled mostly to and the room is filled with a warm fug. The clock ticks slowly on. I rinse my mug out in the sink. I wipe down the surface where a little water's splashed back. I rearrange the lilies. I glance back over towards the Moses basket. And I find myself heading over. I can't stop myself. I peer in and check if he's woken up. He hasn't.

This is my moment. I can do whatever I like. I can let my weary head nod a while on the QT, I can flick through the treasury of nursery stories that someone bought for Jack but which I'm itching to get stuck into, or I can relive my childhood fantasies and perform a Torvill and Dean double-axel pirouette in front of the stove and nobody'd be any the wiser.

But I don't. All I can think of is gazing, mesmerised at the beauty of my child, his tightly curled fingers, his perfectly round downy face, and the gentle rise and fall of his chest. He's breathing. That's a good sign.

His fair colouring and wrinkled frown remind me unmistakably of his dad. His absent dad. This is the way it's going to be son, just you and me. Don't get me wrong, I'm not planning on bumping Daddy off, finding myself suddenly single or doing a runner any time soon. I'm just facing up to the reality of life at home with a small baby while my other half's out working goodness knows where and for goodness knows how long. That's just the way it is. One of life's bummers. Like finding out you've written a song entitled 'Ironic' that in fact proves you don't know what irony means.

Or is it a bummer? The way I'm feeling now I could happily submerge myself into the moment and let go, drifting oblivious to all else gently off into my future. I'm Anne from my own childhood stories, lying in a flat-bottomed boat, lost in my own little play act. I've left the others behind on the shore. I'm lying perfectly still on an old black shawl. My red curls fan out about my head. A tall bloom is placed in folded hands across my breast. It is all that could be desired.

Until the boat springs a leak and cold reality floods back in. The phone starts to ring, Jack starts to cry and an unexpected damp patch has begun to flower across my top. *I* am actually leaking. I'm *properly* producing milk. I feel like cutting off whoever's ringing so I can call the indifferent midwife and rejoice in the fact that my milk's now coming thick and fast.

We're a small but select party, and the drinks are on me!

Charlotte
Thomas & Friends, plus Random Mothers being Driven Round the Bends
Based, roughly, on The Railway Series by the Rev. W. Awdry.

TO THE TRAINS ->

This is a story about Charlotte, a bright red-faced new mummy. Charlotte didn't think she was very special because she only hefted around empty trucks. But one day, Charlotte realised just how useful she was ...

It was a blustery morning on the Island of Arsendor.

'Toot toot,' called Dirk to the stationmaster and puffed off.

Thomas pulled into Blackstock Docks and noticed a new mummy, Charlotte, looking very sad.

'What's the matter?' puffed Thomas.

'I don't feel Very Useful because I'm lugging around empty trucks.'

Just then the signal turned to red. A Community Midwife thundered past with the Express. 'You wait there and stop whingeing,' she chuffed. 'Breast is best. Time to put up and jolly well get on with it!'

Charlotte chugged sadly off.

As Thomas wondered what to do, Charlotte hummed and hawed a bit, muttering 'I don't care what they say,' in a quiet siding. She glanced at her empty trucks wretchedly.

Another midwife chuffed in, and drew to a halt when the stationmaster waved a red flag. 'Try the formula. Try the formula,' she chuntered before puffing quickly away.

Charlotte felt more confused than ever.

Suddenly a big gust of wind blew the tarpaulin covering the trucks off. Charlotte looked around at her trucks again and realised that she *was* carrying round a special load after all, it'd just been hiding that was all.

Charlotte raced off to the yard to tell Thomas the news. 'I feel very special now,' she puffed, a big smile on her face.

'More trucks, more trucks!' called out Dirk whooshing past and off out the station again at high speed.

Without a moment's thought, Charlotte rushed back into the yard. She couldn't wait to get her trucks out again. She was so proud it made her axles tingle.

Charlotte now knew what it was like to feel Really Useful.

I feel at once both jubilant and ever so slightly crackers. I'm an Olympic medallist. I'm a *Pop Idol* vote winner. I'm Mr Happy, fat and yellow with a U-shaped grin. I'm a brainy but photogenic A-Level student on results day snapped mid air-punch for tomorrow's papers. I am Katrina with her Waves and I'm walking on sunshine.

Is it the lack of sleep, my hormones playing ping-pong or the effect of too much coffee too quick after a lengthy caffeine abstinence? Whatever the catalyst, the result is exhilarating. I reckon I could certainly give that Jayne Torvill a run for her money right now if I *but* had a pair of streamline skates to hand. Shame.

The phone persists a little longer and then rings off as I'm lifting the now incandescent Jack out of his basket. I know I'm no expert, but *he* doesn't appear to be walking on sunshine. 'You made me wait three minutes! Three. Whole. Minutes!'

I sink tentatively onto the sofa, my abdomen still stabbing at me meanly if I try to take things too fast. I hush my whimpering child and fiddle with fresh competence at my complicated new feeding bra. It's a clever flippy number with neat plastic gizmos that provide easy one-flick access to what lies beneath. Inspector Gadget surely wore one underneath his brown mackintosh. And surely teenage boys would give their eye teeth to get their hands on a few spotty teenage girls wearing these. In some parts of the country, perhaps they already do.

Flap duly flipped, and ... ahhh ... he's off. Jack goes into auto-pilot, sucking Nature's own pink and malleable gobstopper. I'm only hoping he doesn't try crunching it when he gets to the end.

A wave of love envelops me as I gaze at the side of Jack's head. Those jaws, I reassure myself, are as yet incapable of crunching. Or so I hope. I breathe the sweet intoxicating odour of his scalp, the milky softness of his skin and his unblemished innocence. I'm blown away with unmitigated love. I now understand my own mother's love for me.

The phone begins to ring again. This time I reach over, briefly pulling myself away from my indignant son to pick up the receiver. With an expertise that belies my amateur status, I jam the handset under my chin and plug the searching lips back on as though I've been doing it for years.

'Hello?'

'Hi, Chaz. It's only me. Just thought I'd call and find out how you're getting on?'

'Oh, hi, Mum. I'm fine, thanks. *We're* fine. I think.'

Chapter 9

I twitch the curtain furtively and take a look out. It is another hot sunny day. Dirk's been back at work a while now. Both grandparents have returned home. It's time to pull myself out of the porridge. It's time to go out.

The pile of leaflets the Health Visitor had brought along are staring me accusingly in the face, hurt by my cruel lack of attention. I steel myself, find the one that has been silently beckoning, and then spend half of the morning gazing at it, wondering if I can crack this breastfeeding lark by matter of osmosis. Then Jack starts grizzling again and I figure I can't.

And so I tog us up, amble up the road and get us both to the Health Centre at roughly the time advertised, a small achievement in itself. I chain up my buggy outside with a cycle lock as there's not enough room inside for them all. I hoik out the car seat and bring it in with my sleeping babe inside. I wince at my pulling stitches, at the familiar institutional smell of antiseptic and at the very idea of being here. A breastfeeding support group. Sorry, I've made a big mistake. Can I leave now?

I wonder who exactly will be doing the supporting? And how? I have horrible visions of a kaftaned hippie cupping my breasts in her hands and chanting incantations to the milk god. I'm about to turn heel, step back outside and unchain my buggy sharpish. But it's too late, I've been spotted and I'm now being reeled in.

'Are you here for the breastfeeding group?'

'Erm. Yes. I think so.'

'Righto. Just make your way through the double doors at the back. They've just started. In you go.' Like a crash test dummy, I'm compelled forward to meet my fate behind the double doors.

The first few weeks of adapting to life with my new baby had been a flurry of home-based activity. No DIY to speak of, just a lot of comings and goings through our house while Jack and I trod water on the spot and cried. With the benefit of hindsight and a quick search on the Net, I can now see what I was suffering from.

The Common Holed-Up

WHAT IS THE COMMON HOLED-UP?

Holed-Up is a non-contagious but flummoxing state of inertia which affects nine out of ten new mums. The characteristic symptom is not setting foot outdoors for days. Usually, it is a mild condition, recovery taking place within a couple of weeks. However, sometimes the same symptoms occur with other illnesses like Can't be Bothered Dressingfluenza, in which case, if left unchecked, it may go on for years. Or at least until the Milk Chocolate Digestives run out and you fancy buying a paper.

HOW DO WE DEVELOP 'HOLED-UP'?

A new mummy is prone to hibernate from the day before the baby breaks out until one to three days after they feel better.

The need to retreat is spread by airborne expectations of how to conduct oneself in public with a newborn. It can also be exacerbated if the person is experiencing extreme soreness in their abdomen or other places where the sun don't usually shine.

WHAT ARE THE SYMPTOMS OF HOLED-UP?

- A sore stomach or 'front bottom'. (You're *so* over being nonchalant about naming the rude bits by now.)
- There may be pain on swallowing some of the unsolicited advice.
- Coughing when Community Midwife proposes checking on your stitches.
- Headache when Community Midwife points to baby's jaundice and suggests you should really get out more.
- Eyes beginning to run with a water-like secretion which gradually pours uncontrollably down cheeks at times of duress such as during howling infant's heel prick test, your hormones deciding it's a super day to pogo, or the bread's run out and you've forgotten how to cope.

WHAT CAN YOU DO TO AVOID CATCHING HOLED-UP?

- You may feel like you want to run away but chances are you'll get it anyway, so you might as well just accept it.
- You could try washing your hands thoroughly and avoid touching your nose or eyes after being in physical contact with your new baby. It will do nothing to prevent Holed-Up but at least gives you something to do while you're incarcerated so you might as well, eh.
- Keep rooms well aired. Although not too well aired.

- Remember the risk of freak newborn frostbite if rooms are not tropical at all times.

I'm ushered in and sit down. So far, no head-on collision. A slight woman with curly hair and a brisk manner welcomes us in. 'Your baby is beautiful,' she says looking down into the car seat. I wonder on what basis she's made her judgement, given Jack's still fast asleep and wrapped up in many obscuring layers. Which is how I hope he (and me) will stay. Maybe Jack will sleep on till the end of the session and I'll be let off the hook?

'Oh, I bet you say that to all the girls,' I blather nervously.

'Come on, then. Out you come, sunshine.' She reaches in and pulls off the top blanket.

What? You're going to wake my sleeping baby? The one I spend hours trying to settle and who's peacefully away with the fairies right now. Fairies like Oberon who are helping to keep my Titanias firmly under wraps.

'Here she is,' she says. 'Goodness, she's just a little one. We'll soon have you feeding her properly up, though.'

Jack's disgruntled face creases into an angry crimson knot. I can feel mine following suit. There's a pause. A deep breath. And a fairly sizeable howl for *just a little one.*

How dare she, I think, feeling my face turning as pink as the clothes my son might be wearing if he was a girl. Mistaking his sex I can forgive, however (though Jack's still kicking off about the insult). I'm more cross at the implied criticism of my feeding performance. Have I not been doing enough? Were the hours suckling my ever-hungry baby insufficient? Did my late-night feeding marathons, complete with bleeding nipples and gritted teeth, not go far enough? Was enduring David 'Cheap as Chips' Dickinson daytime TV to get through another feed not already going the extra mile?

Apparently not. My baby is still small. He's been bumping along the bottom of that graph of theirs, bruising his bony bum as blue as the not-pink Babygro he's currently in. I'm told he's not gaining weight fast enough. (Doesn't get that from me. Obviously.) And with the scales still reading well below the Gina starting point, I've been persuaded that attending this comfortable and supportive group might be helpful.

Helpful my (nicely cushioned) bottom. Whoever thought up the 'comfortable and supportive' tag got it wrong then. At the moment I feel I'm being judged and found wanting. It's like a bad appraisal, only worse because I've only had about three hours sleep in the last fortnight.

Why don't you just hand me my P45 right now and have done with it, I think. But instead I croak 'Erm, yes, I think we've been having a few issues.'

'Well, for starters, sit yourself down and pop your baby on this pillow. What I'm hearing right now is a very hungry baby. So let's feed her, shall we?'

'Him. He's a him.'

The photo album cover is orange with black and beige vertical stripes. There are slippery opaque protection leaves between the pages that are now starting to yellow. The pictures are all mounted with neat little sticky triangles.

Inside is a smattering of pictures of my brother, my parents' first-born, a couple of days old. In the hospital fish tank (same as Jack's). Back at home in his gargantuan cot. In his mother's arms in the garden. He's gorgeous. His eyes are tight shut. He's probably trying to shield his eyes from the visual explosion all around that is the 1970s.

Mum's wearing a figure-skimming floral blouse with more browns and oranges than a packet of Jaffa Cakes. She's sitting on a turquoise-patterned sofa. And beside her is a casual side table adorned with a crazy patchwork tablecloth in a kaleidoscope of yet more browns and oranges.

Mum's not looking at the camera, she's too busy gazing at her infant son. Whoever's taken the picture managed to get in a good few inches of Mum's exposed mini-skirted thigh. (Well done, Dad.) He's not, however, managed to get Mum and my brother Ed in focus. Instead, picked out in perfect precision on the side table is a bowl of cotton wool and talcum powder, and a nearly finished bottle of milk.

Ed's wrapped up in a brushed-cotton sheet adorned with cutely dressed chicks and orange-centred daisies. I know the feel of this blanket. As a girl, I used to pop it over my plastic dollies in their pint-sized plastic prams. When I got older and the dollies were left shivering on the shelf, the sheet transferred to the cat's basket where it moulded, warm around her fastidiously clean body. We took her to the vet in that sheet, swaddled and secure. Only the sheet returned home, the yellow chicks now much faded, covered with a fine layer of downy black hair.

I can smell the love on that blanket, still virgin fresh, enfolded round my newborn brother. I can sense Mum's joy and vulnerability. Faded and seventies-tastic, it seems so very far away. But also so close.

She was alone, more alone than I am with my support groups, NCT buddies and quick off the marks visiting grandparents. There *was* her friend Jean, a fellow Brit in Canada and first-time mum. And clinicians on hand in case of crisis. Dad, who returned to work immediately after dropping his wife and newborn back home from hospital, would have been home in the evenings too, though New Man hadn't sprung in on the scene yet. For much of the time, however, there was isolation.

Trying to cope with a demanding newborn. Wilting summer heat. Croup, waiting to pounce just around the corner. No wonder she hit the bottle. Of course in those days formula was the norm and even the fashion. Some things change. Others don't.

I look again at Mum in the picture on the sofa. Part of me wants to slide in beside her and put my arm around her shoulder. She'll get on with it and get through it. But I'm fairly sure that, even outside this early photo she remained for a while a bit blurred at the edges.

I'm in a cosy Victorian terrace in Stoke Newington a few weeks later. Half-drunk mugs rest on the reclaimed pine kitchen table. The kettle's been doing sterling service all morning.

Later, the mugs will be accompanied by plates of rice cakes. The babies will grab hold of one gamely, squishing the saliva-glooped cardboard between their fingers and more often than not down all down their mummies' clothes. There will be pots of milky wallpaper paste (mm!), pulped banana, and obscenely orange carrot and lentil mush. (The nappies thereafter will be historic.) There will also be pots of parental anxiety as the grown-ups stoop to furtive 'is that baby more advanced at eating than mine' progress checks. But we're not quite there yet. The babies are all still pre-solids and contentedly nuzzling into our breasts. Today we're all on a level playing field. Or are we? I don't let on that I've started to give a bottle at night. It feels like my dirty secret. I'm not performing as I should.

The Health Visitor has been practically begging me to top up on my feeds. The weight's still not going on sufficiently in spite of my improved technique. I feel a bit like a pinball. At first I'd shot into the game with barely a backward glance but now I'm being knocked back and forth with confusing speed. I've been clinging to the premise that if I succeed at breastfeeding I'll succeed in being a mum. But a flipper's just caught me at blinding speed from left field and I've been shot up a ramp. The mentors who'd hitherto been banging on about breast being best, and woe to she who doubts it, are now confusingly encouraging me to bring on the formula. I think I'll just disappear down this sinkhole for a bit to think.

So if I persist in exclusively breastfeeding then Jack falls off the weight graph. Below the entire range of averages for the country. Surely that's impossible? But if I agree to top up with bottles his weight is likely to pick up, I'll get more than two hours' sleep at a time and I'll get to self-flagellate at every turn. How's that for a can't-refuse offer?

I really didn't want to throw in the towel. I saw it as an admission of failure. Dirk wanted me to throw the bottle in the steriliser, however, and buck up a bit because he wanted the smiling version of his wife back. Not the waxwork model version with a pallid face and hair that's not quite right, but the real McCoy again.

Someone tilts the pinball machine and it's game over. I start to top up my feeds with formula and I start to claw back my sanity. I sleep for three-hour stretches for the first time in an eternity. Jack starts to gain weight and gets dimples. The days turn into weeks. My son learns to smile. And so, again, do I.

At around 16–20 weeks your baby may show signs of being ready for his or her first taste of solids. You can start off gently, and then quickly progress to an all-out taste 'n' waste bonanza. Try some of the following in your baby's feeds and let the real fun and games begin.

LENTILS

Adding lentils to a baby puree provides a good source of fibre, adding a bit of explosive fun to your otherwise fairly dull nappy-changing routine. You can be sure that introducing lentils is a sure-fire way of making his nappy, the changing mat and your bathroom floor resemble the infamous Wreck of the Hesperus. (Note to the novice; do not, whatever you do, feel tempted to change your baby's nappy on the bed after feeding it lentils.)

CARROTS

Carrots also make excellent weaning food because of their naturally sweet taste and, teamed with the lentils, will provide nuclear-inspired colour variation to changing times.

SWEET POTATOES AND BUTTERNUT SQUASH

You've probably never cooked these guys before, and perhaps never yet had the occasion to hobnob at all, but if you add them to your shop, the checkout assistant will *know* you're cooking on gas when it comes to feeding bubs.

SWEETCORN

Don't even go there.

Feeding the five thousand, well OK, just the three of them turns out of course to be far trickier than bunging lentils down a lone baby's mush, notwithstanding the explosive results.

The demands of my three growing boys turn out to be much more complex. My own demands are too. I want, quite reasonably I think, to:

a) keep their tastes reasonably adventurous
b) model their eating habits on our own so that they end up eating roughly the same diet as us
c) cook something that takes minimal preparation so when it's rebuffed I don't feel I've wasted another three hours of my life (Hell after all hath no fury than a mummy whose laboriously made fish pie has been rejected)

So here I am, sitting at the kitchen table, flicking through Nigel Slater's *Real Fast Food*, looking for inspiration. I like the idea of fast. Fast is good. But I'm rubbish at recipe books without pictures. I like to know what to expect, what I'm aiming to plonk on the plate at the end of my quick multi-speed cheffing sesh. Or at least have an idea of how to present it (parsley just like so, and so on and so forth).

But no, my paperback's just text with a couple of namby-pamby line drawings of unpeeled garlic cloves and whole shiny aubergines. I know what my raw ingredients look like. I need to be shown what they *could* look like given the right handling.

I flip past Hot Mussels in Curry Cream and Mackerel Teriyki. Don't think those will pass muster with the junior diners. I'm not chancing anything too elaborate any more. Ah. Here we have it, a 'Better Egg Sandwich', a 'Fish Finger Sandwich' or 'Rumblede-thumps'. If you look closely enough there's sure to be an answer lurking somewhere. I have no idea what Rumbledethumps are but the name should sell it to them, though if it takes a second longer than the promised thirty minutes and they *still* refuse it I shall of course go around and throw a rotten egg at Nige's window. (I know what an egg looks like. There are two of them helpfully drawn out in pencil for me on page 49. It's unclear how I'd tell if they were rotten but I'd be willing to chance it.)

* * *

Further along in the same family photo album, there's a picture of Mum and Dad with an older baby Ed. Dad's matured a bit since his wedding day. He now looks about fourteen but he's wearing a tie that looks suspiciously like it should belong in school and that doesn't help.

Mum's looking young and relaxed. Her hair's a little shorter. She's holding her beautifully turned-out son up with a confident double-handed grasp as if to say to their distant families back home: 'Here's one for the album. Isn't he big and healthy. We've managed. Haven't we done well?'

I for one am impressed. From the look of Dad's forward tilt and his left arm stretching out of shot towards the camera he's taken the picture himself. And he's managed to get this one in focus.

Autumn. There is a definite 'back to school' chill in the air. Spiders are spinning their webs at head height, doing their utmost to catch you in the ghost train horror of sticky stuff in your hair. Fireworks are going off at random times of day and night. Shop windows are turning black and orange. Life is returning to normality.

I've got a little routine going on now. Nothing like the hour-by-hour efficient drill Gina would have had me follow, but a comforting weekly whirl of toddler groups, baby music and wrapped-up potters round the park. I now am one of those perambulating mummies I watched from that park bench not so very long ago.

These days I walk and walk for Britain. Heels have been swapped for sensible flats as I pound the local streets and parks. I discover passageways and open spaces that I didn't know existed. I stray into de Beauvoir, Mildmay and Stoke Newington. I pop into local shops to pick up a pint of milk, an exchange of pleasantries and wide smiles and thank-yous as the doors are held ajar to allow me and the buggy out.

It's a far cry from air-conditioned offices, automatic Tube doors, little in the way of eye contact. I now feel I belong. I'm part of the community. It's no longer just about me starting to recognise regular faces. I am also one of the faces too.

I push the buggy down Church Path on the way to Highbury Fields where I'd stealthily watched the mummies I was set to join. A corridor of mature chestnut trees lines the route and it's Russian roulette when the conkers start to drop. I pull the hood up over Jack's exposed face.

It's still quite mild. A couple of tracksuited tennis players are whacking a ball back and forth over the net in the courts nearby. The Oasis Café is drawing in those in search of coffee, a sit-down and a plate of aubergines, their kids begging for unseasonal ice creams. A jogger runs past, headphones on, listening, maybe, to the strains of 'Dilemma' (shall I pick up that coffee now or later?).

I hurry past them on the way to Baby Music. We'll be leaving Nelly and Kelly to their indecision and singing 'Horsey Horsey' and 'Going to the Zoo' instead. I say *we'll* be singing but technically Jack won't be doing much trilling. I'll do the singing while I bounce him, baffled, on my lap. As well as fitting in a bit of essential chit-chat with my mates.

This of course invokes a barrage of tut-tutting from the guitar-strumming leader who'd prefer us all to take it all a bit more seriously. *She* takes it extremely seriously. There's her table of instruments that the kids are warned in no uncertain terms to steer well clear of. There's her stash of coloured ribbons which we're urged to flutter around to the music, a challenge when said ribbons are often grabbed, scrunched and swiftly weighted down with the goo of fresh saliva. And there's her bag of sweeties, which I presume she dips into in order to keep her vocal cords comfortably lubricated. Either that or it's a comfort thing as she realises the roomful of yakking mummies are cheerfully ignoring her and chatting over her entreaties to join in with the tickly caterpillar song.

At the end, she tries reeling us back in with some Beatles or Mamas and Papas as though they'll encourage us to Let our chatting Be and stop Highbury Dreaming in favour of concentrating on the serious matter in hand.

But the whole point is, the key matter *is* about us chatting. I'm not here to teach Jack all the lines to Old MacDonald and expect him to rattle them off verbatim and perfectly in tune by the end of the term. I'm here to network through song. Meet up with other mummies. Cement the tentative friendships that are just beginning to flower.

It's a Thursday after school, a few years on. 'Going to the Zoo' feels like an age ago. The boys are in paradise. Late afternoon sun streams in through the glazed kitchen door, perfectly highlighting the selection of grubby handprints arranged in random clots on the smeary glass. I make a mental note to call the window cleaner. A mischievous grin is flowering across Billy's face. Jack is standing on his chair. Sid thumps a yoghurty spoon on the table and our guest, Luke, is saying nothing.

We're in the middle of a tea date. The sofa has already been pulled apart and made into a rocket ship with a slide. The Lego bucket has been upturned on the floor and abandoned. The dressing-up clothes are strewn willy-nilly all down the stairs, a multicoloured waterfall of fun.

We've just finished eating tea. Jack has dined in a doctor's coat, stethoscope dangling from his neck. Luke is Peter Pan. Billy *was* a cowboy but lost his Stetson somewhere en route to his sausages. Sid is the audience, no costume as such, but there's now a thick layer of Petits Filous concealing a fair part of his face.

Billy is grinning like Paul Newman when Redford's told him he can't swim. Jack is still tottering on the chair, ready for a blast.

'Do you want to hear our cool song?' he says, keen to show off.

Not waiting for the response, he reaches for the CD case and pulls out the shiny silver disc. It annoys me when he does that. The next time he puts it on and there's a scratch who'll come complaining to me? It will of course be all my fault.

Today I leave him to it though, not wanting to cramp his style. He grabs the remote and selects play, more savvy with the gadgets than I will ever be. Jack and Billy launch delightedly together into their song.

'This is the best bit ... "We will, we will rock you!"'

Pause accompanied by two contented smirks.

'"We will, we will rock you!"'

Furtive sideways glances at each other. Enormous grins. Fervent handclaps, not necessarily the sequence to fit the song but they're loving it anyway. They make an odd couple. They look like a pair of novices at aerobics, earnestly trying to keep up, but making a complete hash of it. They look not, as Jack had suggested, remotely cool in front of the mate they're trying to impress. They look, to be honest, pretty silly.

The chorus comes back around again. There's a pause. Billy and Jack look at Luke earnestly. And then Luke joins in the crazy handclap routine, laughing. Sid giggles uncontrollably. They are rocking along just fine.

The mummies all went in one by one, apart, apart.
The mummies all went in one by one, apart, apart.

The mummies all went in one by one, but they went back
   again so as not to feel shunned,
And they *all* went to this sing-along lark, for to feel
   human again.

The mummies all went in two by two, hurrah, hurrah.
The mummies all went in two by two, hurrah, hurrah.
The mummies all went in two by two, 'Nice to meet you,
   and to meet you too,'
And they *all* left for a play in the park, for to feel human
   again.

The mummies all went in three by three, hurrah, hurrah.
The mummies all went in three by three, hurrah, hurrah.
The mummies all went in three by three, 'D'ya fancy
   having a cup of tea?'
And they *all* left for a char in the park, for to feel human
   again.

The mummies all went in four by four, hurrah, hurrah.
The mummies all went in four by four, hurrah, hurrah.
The mummies all went in four by four, 'Same again, my
   place or yours?'
And they *all* left for a goss and a laugh, for to feel human
   again.

It's a weekday lunchtime in December. I'm wedged in behind a stuffed-to-capacity restaurant table on Islington Green. We are here to enjoy a festive jolly and let our hair down a bit. Well for as long as we can stand having it grabbed and yanked by our juvenile dates, that is.

Jack's squirming excitedly on my knees, determined to bring

the contents of the table in for closer inspection. The cutlery and glassware get pushed periodically about like model submarines on a military planning map. It's all about strategic timing, and well-executed shoves in order to avoid getting a knife, a plate of food or the whole cascading tablecloth drawn onto your lap.

We're all here, my NCT gang, and it's our self-appointed company 'Christmas do'. Why miss out on all the fun just because you're not in an office? It's the time of year to have fun, relax and enjoy. But just in case anyone's got any daft ideas up their sleeves, we've set out a few guidelines before things start getting silly.

NCT Girls' Crimbo Party Dos and Don'ts

- People can get overexcited and may act out of character at Christmas parties. Everyone today is to remain sensible and just be themselves (apart from the guy who's drafted in to play Santa. Sorry, did I spoil it for you?).
- No photocopying of bottoms for a laugh, we've all seen quite enough of those already this year.
- No disappearing into broom cupboard for a bit of how's your father. This is strictly a 'No daddies' do.
- Health and Safety have made a review of the tinsel, tree and fairy-light set-up and deemed them all well out of curious little fingers' reach. So no whingeing, OK?
- All mummies are to show up for duty tomorrow, absolutely no excuses.

My NCT group is a jolly good bunch even though I say so myself. There's me and Jack, Avril and Scarlett and the rest of the mob and their little ones.

We'd met and instantly bonded, contravening all the Really Important website rules about meeting new contacts. We'd rendezvoused in a private home (though abstained from the hotel room or anywhere remote. You can't find 'remote' in Highbury). We tried to keep our meetings secret but there was no way the neighbours *couldn't* hear us through the walls even without the aid of a glass cup. We let each other know our home addresses almost immediately, and were in and out of each other's houses all the time. And we cavalierly allowed our drinks to be tampered with. 'You put an extra sugar in my tea? Oh, you're *terrible*, that'll do nothing for my hips.'

We soon felt comfortable and safe in each other's company, sharing and baring it all. We compared notes on steaming, skinning and pureeing green beans (verdict = don't bother). We sucked our teeth en masse on whether to jab or not to jab, or whether it was best simply not to question. And we went in safe groups to Baby Massage where the clearly bonkers teacher would warble through 'Getting to Know You' whilst we kneaded and waxed our wriggling charges, getting to know them and their discharges a little too well when she encouraged us to throw caution to the wind, discard their nappies and indulge in a bit of naked, and frequently soggy, upper thigh action.

We spent daylight hours pairing our babes off, comparing and contrasting their names to the daft celebrity newborns (Damian? Rudy? Romeo, anyone?), and we set about plotting ways to escape our offspring. We spend months, some of us years trying to conceive a baby. And then once they're there, we can't wait for time out. Clutch back the illusion of childlessness just for a bit. And where better to start than with a good girls' night at the pub? 'There you are, darling. Baby's asleep in bed. You should be fine. Won't be long. Honest ...'

At this particular jolly, however, we have condescended to bringing our children with us. The Christmas babes-on-lap lunch affair would, however, be the last of its kind. Novices that we were, we had made a basic mistake in a party that involved children which we would never make again.

Dining tables and children's parties don't mix. Not in the usual manner of use. Any party involving children of *any* age does not involve sitting around a table. On it, under it, dancing around it, maybe. But not sitting civilised around it. Because kids are like those delayed-action springing toys. The ones with a plastic pirate, an animal or a spherical smiley face on top. You push them down onto the coiled rubber suction pad. Wait for a bit, breath baited. A little longer perhaps? And then – you always knew it was coming – up they jump! There's just no way of keeping them down!

Never expect to sit for long.

A couple of mouthfuls of linguine down and we think it's all over. It is now.

It all begins with the clatter of a knife onto the floor. Someone's taken their eye off the ball and one of the submarines has been captured. A set of keys are dangled in a bid for distraction, but these babies are nobody's fool. Who wants keys when you could have that nice shiny pepper mill? An undercurrent of dissent begins to bubble. First one breaks into tears and then the others follow.

Those who are still breastfeeding clamp their wailing babes on. I fish desperately into my bag for the formula. Technically speaking, Jack's not due for a feed yet, but there's no way he's taking a Whoozit for an answer. I snip and pour the ready-made packet of SMA Gold into the pre-sterilised bottle. I screw the lid back on, to a mounting crescendo on my lap. I tip the bottle and push the teat towards the now frantic lips. And then he spits it back out at me in disgust.

He continues to shriek all the while that the bottle is being spirited to and from the kitchen microwave. The waitress had taken it away with Basil Fawlty disdain after I'd asked her to heat it for me, just a little. 'How dare you try to fob me off with cold milk,' Jack is remonstrating, loudly. To the other diners it just sounds like a baby who's livid with his mother and who should, really, be removed from the restaurant asap. Out of sight, out of mind and most importantly out of earshot. To me it sounds like a pre-emptive strike against the waitress for tardy service.

When she finally returns, it becomes apparent that not only is she slow, she also intends to burn the roof off the mouth of the screaming wailer who is disturbing the peace. She hands over the bottle. It is hot as molten lava. She gives me a 'That should get rid of the riff raff' smile and turns heel. I get up, taking my screaming baby, my scalding bottle and my harried expression with me. I've worked out it might be prudent to temporarily leave the building.

I'd always been a good girl. I got the grades at school. I fought doggedly through my degree with my schoolgirl French amongst people who'd been brought up bilingually. I set my sights on a career that would tick the boxes. I was never going to be the doctor Mum had hoped for, but I wasn't going to be knocking around selling ripped-off designer handbags off a market stall either. (No disrespect to the Del Boys of the Chanel-accessories world.)

I met and married a respectable chap. He brushed up well and charmed Mum with an outsize bunch of flowers. He gained my dad's respect by matching him pint for pint in the pub. He swept me off my feet when doing so would not incur a long-term back injury and we were duly married. I was twenty-two, the same age as my mum when she'd got wed.

We married in St Mary Magdalene's in a village near

Cambridge. It is a beautiful and timeworn church whose congregation had warmly welcomed us in as one of their number. I'd won a bridal magazine competition and scooped the dress, a sparkly white number with a daftly long train; morning suit for the groom, the best man and the Father of the Bride; use of a vintage car for the day which turned the men into wide-eyed little boys. Their gapes provided free entertainment for everyone else. It was a beautiful day in spite of the dark skies. Happy is the bride the rain falls on. And I was. Rained on and happy. Everything was as it should be.

So far, so conventional.

Time progressed. I grew up in my marriage and started doing proper grown-up things like reading the Sunday papers, listening to Frank Sinatra, contributing to a mortgage and getting a proper job. As opposed to those improper murky student jobs of yore. I hadn't seen anything wrong with dragging random people off the street into nearby hotels *per se* but I didn't ultimately see my future in Market Research, quizzing folk on their cream cheese-buying preferences or how they rated the prototype Domestos bleach ad.

I'd set my eyes on greater things. I stuck my foot at the bottom of the publishingy, marketingy type ladder and began to climb. I'd never particularly had clear direction on what I wanted to be when I grew up, nor was I especially ambitious. So I just gently set off, meandering on a course of discovery accumulating experience, different-coloured payslips and Keep your Feet on the Ground Miles. That's Air Miles on a bike or in a Renault 5.

I worked in shiny new out-of-town business complexes and old-town higgedly-piggedly characterful holes. I'd sold Poison and cashmere jumpers, and issued library fines. I'd tinkered with HMSO egg statistics, scabies and Bradford Students' Union.

I'd dipped into a bit of French rosacée, Concorde and the new Millennium. I'd worked in and around London, Paris, Cambridge, Huntingdon and Harlow, a rich set of locations most of which have been captured in oils at some point by one or more of the best-loved Impressionists. (I don't care what anyone says, to me it's clear as day that Monet's *Impression, Soleil Levant* is set on the River Lea and the boat's just popped up from Enfield Lock that morning.)

It may have seemed a bit haphazard. Ah, who am I trying to kid, I was all over the place. But it all contrived to fill up my CV and make me look busy. And I genuinely wasn't sitting on my laurels as I eventually jumped into the surf and caught the multimedia wave. Where Mum had in her time been at the forefront of ultrasound-scanning technology, I was up there and clinging on to CGI scripts, jpegs and metatags for all my worth.

Don't think I was all clever about it. I'm as technical as a teacup. But I was a pretty good project manager, even though I say so myself. The secret of my success was to write everything down. I'd write down and confirm telephone conversations by email. I'd scribble copious meeting notes with large circled CMs to remind me of my many action points. And in the midst of a demanding conference call I'd stick a Post-it note on my monitor scrawled 'Go to loo'.

Lists were my thing. There'd be the work-to-do list ranging from 'get new Post-its from stationery cupboard' to 'book flight to Harare (if airline still flying there)'; the shopping list ('Slim-a-Soup', 'meals for one'); and somewhere gathering dust the New Year resolutions list ('I *will* learn to parallel park', 'I *will* lose a stone').

I'd cross out items done in bold felt tip, though invariably the to-dos still outnumbered the dones. I'd retrospectively write in previously unaccounted-for things done and then cross them straight out to make myself feel better.

Was I trying to achieve a sense of control amidst the burgeoning demands on my time? Was I just delaying getting on with the job in hand by pretending to be supremely organised? Or was I just trying to prove my self-worth by consigning to paper the proof of how I spent my days?

My last professional KPIs were all about team leading and process development. It was about organising people to publish online information that would ultimately help others organise their travel. Ironic, given the rather haphazard path I'd felt I'd taken to get here. But was it and was I?

Surely underneath I only got to where I was because I'd built up the experience and confidence to do my job and do it well? I'd variously picked up manager, leader and executive tags throughout my professional meanderings so I can't have been all that bad. Admittedly 'executive' is one of those ambiguous labels that's often applied to random things to make them sound a bit more attractive. Like 'executive desk' = MDF table with a couple of drawers and room for an anglepoise, available separately, or 'executive lunch' = a shiny oval plate of limp sandwiches around a meeting room table with a glass of the ubiquitous Hillingdon Spring water on the side.

But I refuse to believe I was only given the executive bit because I was like a cheap piece of office furniture that needed glamorising. I was and am, in fact, rather expensively put together with a couple of reconstructed teeth, a regular paint job at the hairdressers and an outlay of well in excess of £3.50 each month on clothes.

Apart from the titles, I had a stack of decent appraisals under my belt, a team of colleagues who appeared to appreciate me and even a plea to stay when I was offered another job closer to home that would be an end to my daft commute. They must've rated me. And I guess I felt comfortable. Needed. Wanted. Performing as expected.

And then I threw it all up like a deck of cards to be at home with my children.

Jack is nine months old. It is technically the end of my maternity leave. I'm typing up my verbally agreed application for extended unpaid leave. I've decided to prolong my stint at home, spending time with my baby and immersing myself in the cosy fug of blending cooked veg, hanging damp vests on the radiators and changing legions of squidgy nappies. I'm casting aside my professional hat and clinging resolutely to the sou'wester of motherhood instead.

(I tell you, every kit list of what to buy when you become a mum should include one. It is impossible to push a buggy and hold a brolly at the same time, so invest in a good rain hat. Do it, if you do nothing else.)

I've changed, not only in my headwear, but in more ways than I care to think of over this last nine months. I'm a different person to the one who stashed the Winnie the Pooh bag into my car all that time ago. I will, without doubt, change again.

If you're looking for the queen of reinvention, then look no further than my mum. I'm not suggesting she's had more hairstyles than Madonna but boy, has she done stuff.

Back through the mists of nearly forty years, she met and married a chap who would take pleasure in claiming to be disrespectable. He had a Heathcliff mop of dark hair, a penchant for a pint and a growling Mustang convertible. My earliest memories were of a classic seventies fashion victim, renouncing all style as far as I could tell and embracing the look of a tramp with brown slacks, a heavy sheepskin jacket and facial hair that would've terrified even Bluebeard. But Mum saw promise in him, the young and fresh-faced scientist who would put the world to rights with his research into glass technology. She saw a man with whom she could share life's ups and downs, and one with whom she could build a home. She also saw a man who respected her for what she was and what she did, her quest to go out into the world and make something of herself. The blonde hair and good legs had absolutely nothing to do with it.

Like me, she grew up in her marriage. Upon this she built up her career and sense of self-worth. She followed a different path though. She went through dark rooms and strip-lit rooms. She worked both by day and at night. She covered all bases. She just did things differently. The wrong way round.

In her day things were different, especially for girls. There was no expectation of furthering your education or of university. She might've liked to but it just wasn't the way. So she left school at sixteen. Got a traineeship and then a job in the NHS after qualifying in radiography. She gained in experience and rank. She had children. She quickly returned to work, needs must. She branched into Ultrasound. She stopped work to sample stay-at-home motherhood, which she briefly did on top of learning to swim when I was about nine. Then she did the education bit. She got a degree as a mature student from Cambridge. She got an MA. Then another one. (It was so good she MAed it twice.) Not to be stopped there, she did a PhD. Before immersing herself into others' education, employed by Cambridge University. And then quitting that in order to put what she had learned back into ongoing learning in the university of the NHS. Its goal was to promote excellence within the NHS.

She's reinvented herself so many times that it's enough to make you dizzy. She's a self-made woman and I take my hat off to her. She's worked hard for every ounce of her success and I'm immensely proud of her.

And then there's me. I had it all easy, laid on a plate. Private school, university, fluky career moves and a family supporting me all along the way. She brought me up to believe in myself, fly the flag for womankind and take the opportunities that come my way. Sadly, I don't think she meant grabbing the chance to hand in my P45, reacquaint myself with the blender and spend my days cleaning mustardy bottoms with Aloe-scented wipes which will forever remind me of poo.

Of course, setting myself up in a solid and happy marriage followed by the inevitable patter of tiny feet is no big deal. It's been all part of the conventional path after getting a degree and a respectable job under my belt. But not going *back* to work afterwards. Now there's the hiccup.

I had been merrily cantering along, enjoying the rush of working life. Then I fell off. Intentionally. They say that to confront your fears you have to climb straight back on again. But I didn't. I found plenty of fears to tackle by staying right where I was, scrabbling around on the ground for a while. Then I pulled myself together, dusted myself off and got back into the saddle. Only on a different mount. The full-time motherhood mount.

And from where I see it right now, I don't fundamentally care much for the old horse any more. I have forgotten what it feels like. I am too busy relishing the risks, the challenges and the derring-do that come along with my new ride. There are still the odd crash-landings. But when it works, it is magic.

Training for Motherhood on the Job – Non-Accredited Course

FEEDBACK FORM

Feedback given by: Charlotte Moerman, Course Survivor
Date: April 2003

Course Summary:
The Training for Motherhood on the Job course was developed by Sink or Swim Training Consultants. They can't claim all the glory. It's a concept approximately ninety per cent of first-time new mums have dabbled in, with the exception of those that:
- reaped the benefit of having helped mother their younger sibs
- had the foresight to train themselves as Norland Nannies
- just happen to be perfectly naturally gifted at motherhood (cows)

Course Objectives:
Delegates will have learned to hit the ground running. Basically, they didn't have much choice.

Time:
At the time of writing, it seems to have been going on for ever. (What, has it only been nine months?)

Participants:
Just the mother and her newborn. (Luckily I didn't score twins.)
Father has been supportive but largely absent.

Cast of friends has been around and about, but this course was targeted at Mum.

Debrief:

A) Analyse how you *feel* at the end of this nine-month period. Summarise below by completing the sentence 'Right now I feel ...
   - hard in places I never did before. (So *this* is what it feels like to be Pamela Anderson. And without surgery!)
   - surprisingly grateful that my nipples have now developed rhino hide. (Nobody warned me at the start that I was breeding a piranha.)
   - tired. Nay, *really, really* tired.

B) Recap what actually happened during this training period? Recall the most important events and list them chronologically:
   - Baby arrives.
   - Mother falls in love hook, line and sinker.
   - Mother changes identity – different clothes, outlook and even her name.
   - Mother finds that she often talks to herself. There was:
     > 'To BF or not to BF, that is the question.'
     > 'What a piece of work is a mum!'
     and
     > 'All the world's a page, probably in a Gina book.'
   - Mother realises she's survived the storm against all odds but is still pondering whether she finds herself in a comedy or a tragedy.

C) Analyse what you have *learned* during this period. Summarise below by completing the sentence 'I have learned ...

- the existence of a vegetable called 'butternut squash'. I still find it a pig to skin, but I *could* now pick it out in an identity parade.
- that disposable nappies have a front and back. That's why there's a handy picture on one side. (What, you thought they were for the *kids*?)
- that swimming nappies are trickier. (Which twit decided to decorate both sides?)
- the *true* meaning of multitasking – e.g., I can sing all the words to 'Incy Wincy Spider' *and* do the tricky limber-finger actions *at the same time*!
- that it impossible to achieve perfection. Even with Pammy breasts.

D) How do you think this relates back to your work life? How might you apply the principles learned in a professional capacity?
- Erm. Maybe I could offer Natalie from LACAR a banana and avocado mash in recompense for again delaying that Argentinian job? Or a butternut squash one if it's critical?

E) What next? What actions will you take on the back of this exercise? How do you want to apply this learning going forward?
- Oh, I know, I know! I'll get pregnant again!

Chapter 10

We're back at the Elizabeth Garrett Anderson. It's February 2004. I'm flicking through the Sunday papers on a familiar candlewick bedspread. Yellow again. Same, same. It's just me and Dirk and a luxuriously spread-out newspaper. Jack is back at home with my parents, waiting for news. We're all waiting, in fact.

I'm mildly uncomfortable, but I could get quite used to this. Quiet. Dirk to myself. The freedom to read the Sunday paper from cover to cover without interruption, hesitation, repetition or deviation. I read practically everything. The usual. The Appointments section. The ads for conservatories, coach tours around the Tyrol and elasticated, breathable 'slacks'. I consider reading Sport.

I've spent the last five minutes poring over an ad for innovative recliners, which apparently provide a unique headrest, neck and lumbar support that 'automatically synchronise gently as you recline'. They look, in my opinion, fairly ugly. But boy, don't they sound good? Bond must surely have reclined in one of these on his day off.

There's a choice of three. I play the game you do sometimes, where you pick the one that you'd most likely buy yourself. The answer of course would normally be none, but I'm strangely drawn to the green faux-leather one. I turn the page, moving swiftly on. Phew, that was a close one. I scared myself for a minute there.

My pregnancy has been different this time. I've not been commuting back and forth to Heathrow, for starters. I've not been seeking out daily fixes from *The Dorling Kindersley Pregnancy Question and Answer Book* ('Look, Dirk, it says this week the eyelashes are developing!') and I've not been able to nod off at will when that overwhelming tiredness creeps on. You can't when you've got a demanding toddler at your feet. I tried. He prodded me awake. Every time.

I have, however, been gifted with a different level of support this time. Not of the green faux-leather variety. And not by colleagues most of whom, with all due respect, wouldn't know one end of the baby from another (unless it had recently eaten lentils in which case there's no mistaking).

Nope. This pregnancy, I'm pleased to report, has been happily cheered along by my swathe of new mummy friends. Most are sympathetic, like Avril, herself expecting my future godson Luka around the same time as me. Some can barely conceal their horror. (She's left *how* long between babies?)

There once was a girl and she had a whirl at conceiving
    some years after she'd wed.
The first time was good, it went just as it should.
The next it was *radically* quicker.

When we found out I was pregnant again, it was a different affair from last time. We knew what we were doing. This time it was child's play. It was simple as a game of noughts and crosses in fact. We had the white-lidded plastic pencil thingummy (tick). We had the paper in the form of tissues, useful for any eventuality (tick). All we needed next was a nought or a cross in the box. Or a thin blue line to be precise. There it is: whoopee! (Blimey!)

It is fair to say there were fewer bangers and firecrackers this time. Fewer stagey air punches. Fewer elated yells of 'I'm the daddy, almost.' We didn't want to wake up Jack for starters, to have him forever associate the news of an impending new sibling with both his parents appearing to have gone completely bonkers.

For all our mature response this time round, though, we were no less overjoyed. No less dewy-eyed. No less euphoric. Just calmer. Which is ironic really considering how things turned out.

My waters broke as I ran Jack's Saturday night bubbly bath. At first there was a trickle. Was I imagining it? Had I wet myself? Had Jack engineered some gravity-defying splash back? I wondered out loud to Dirk if something was up. He said 'Shall I get a towel?' and then, seeing my face, 'If you think it's coming, call your mum.' I called Mum.

She said '*You can't be.*' There was another indisputable trickle. The hospital advised coming in for a check. It was time to plug the flow of my parents' Valentine's Day meal and bottle of red. They drove to London at breakneck speed. They arrived, we kissed and I climbed into the passenger seat of our new family-sized car to make our way to hospital. I gushed over the new upholstery. Dirk was really chuffed about that.

On the approach to the labour ward reception desk I had another spurt for luck, giving the floor a thoroughly good watering in. (Alan would have been proud.)

'Erm, I think my waters are breaking.'

'Sunshine. Your membranes have well and truly left the building. Let's get you into room 5 and have a good look.'

Ten warm gallons, gushing like Vic Falls
Ten warm gallons, gushing like Vic Falls
And if one extra gallon should accidentally fall (all over
    the passenger seat)
There'll be stains with history, must give Autosheen a
    call.

Upon examination it turns out I'm not in labour as such. I just have a case of Preterm Prelabour Ruptured Membranes, which sounds like a cross between a party political broadcast and an excerpt from an Indiana Jones movie. Only now that I have 'drained', much less exciting and arguably more worrying.

No one is about to raid a tomb or wag their finger at Tony. All I can do now is sit tight, bide my time and play a waiting game. Patients, anyone?

I am being kept in because at only thirty-five weeks my baby born now will be technically premature. Most babies, I'm told, arrive within twenty-four hours of the waters breaking. If I don't go into spontaneous within those all-important twenty-four hours, it is likely that tomorrow I will be whisked back into theatre for another caesarean to prevent the risk of infection. It seems that the baby will arrive by hook or by crook, one way or another soon. We just don't yet know how or when.

I lay the Culture section back on the bed and walk down the stairwell to ground and up again for the tenth time today. Dirk ambles companionably beside me. It's as though we are convivially strolling *la passeggiata* together. Here we go again, promenading the flight of stairs, encouraging our *bambini* to make haste down the appropriate passageway before the clock strikes Monday morning and the surgeon pulls on his latex gloves for the day.

* * *

Jack, one day, ridicules the short legs and slow pace of his younger brother Billy, who replies, laughing like the knowing tortoise: 'Though you are a bit taller than me and don't half show off about it too, I will beat you in a race.' Jack, believing his assertion to be simply impossible, assents to the proposal; and they agree that Mummy should choose the course and fix the goal.

On the day appointed for the race the two start off together. Billy never for a moment stops, but goes on with a single-minded steady galumph straight to the finishing line at the end of the garden. Jack trips over a carelessly left-around scooter lying dangerously by the wayside (now how did that get there?) He falls flat on his nose and starts remonstrating 'It's not fair.'

At last he gets up again, a bit huffy and hacked off. He sets off, moving fast as fast as he can but alas sees that Billy has reached the goal where he is waggling his fingers next to his ears and blowing a raspberry.

Now I am in no way, shape or form implying that Billy beat Jack in the great race to come out of my tummy. That would be nothing short of a miracle given the order of conception. It was true that Billy's sperm and egg partnership in the making had said a polite 'after you' when it came to hitting the bull's eye that would in due course make their host look like a fully fledged darts champion. Thereafter, however, the fruit of their union has never been long to hang around.

Billy is usually most keen to out-trump his bigger brother – in the sweetest, healthiest sibling rivalry way – whenever humanly possible. Like overtaking him in shoe size. Like learning to whistle first. Like undercutting his gestation period. Why hang around in the original Great Escape Race when there's so much to see and do out there?

* * *

I do not necessarily want to give birth to a premature baby. But I certainly do not want another caesarean if I can help it (I think). This means that I need to go into natural labour PDQ if I possibly can.

According to the venerable old wives who know about these things, there are many ways that spontaneous labour can be brought on. These include:

- lots of sex
- eating pineapple and/or liquorice but at a guess I'd say not simultaneously
- acupuncture
- having a sweep – in case of doubt, we're not talking chimneys
- a good hot curry
- raspberry leaf tea
- walking around a lot (up and down stairs optional)
- composing an arm-length 'to-do' list of must-complete urgent jobs
- going somewhere you'd die a death of mortification were you to suddenly and very publicly give birth
- sending your other half away somewhere distant:
  - kayaking up the Amazon
  - trekking up Mount Kilimanjaro
    or
  - getting an early night in back at home in Highbury, just say

I do not plump, unsurprisingly given my current location, for the first option.

Labour and Emergency Procedures

There is understandably some concern amongst novices about

taking part in a plan to assist in the evacuation of a mother, especially one who is undergoing VBAC (birth the way Nature intended) after a cut-on-the-dotted-line job. Mothers who have previously had a caesarean delivery, particularly an elective one, may have:

a) not gone into natural labour before.
b) not – if she's now going into *early* labour – had time to reread her dusty NCT 'Managing Labour' notes from last time. (Oops. Or double oops if she frittered valuable swotting time reading crummy newspaper ads.)
c) heard all sorts of labour horror stories from other mummy friends saying 'I felt like I was dying', 'I'm *never* going to do that again' and 'I told my OH where to ram his box of Scrabble when he suggested a game to take my mind off the pain.'

This type of procedure may be further complicated should the mother's other half have already left the building. Especially if labour, when it finally decides to start, comes quick and dirty.

Action in the Event of a Sprint to the Finish Labour

If you notice a mum-to-be patently in agony or unable to even look at the contraction belt, you should immediately raise the alarm by calling a porter, getting hold of a wheelchair that she will probably refuse to sit in anyway and escorting her down to the labour ward PDQ. The alarm is a low continuous moan, accompanied by flashing eyeballs.

Telephone equipment is provided at Sister's desk and should be used immediately if said mum-to-be appears to have sent her OH home. It should only be used after the Entenox rescue services have been called in, but should not by any account be forgotten about. Not ever. *Jamais*. No excuses.

If telephone equipment *has* been temporarily overlooked and said mum-to-be is all of a sudden on the point of actually delivering her baby, only those trained in Health and Safety procedures should make the call to her husband.

'Hello? Mr Moerman?'

'Ugh. Yes?'

'You'd better get yourself here, your wife is having the baby.'

'Oh, she's finally started has she?'

'Just come. She's *having* it. Now!'

One contraction, two contraction, three contraction, four.

Five contraction, six contraction, seven contraction, roar.

One contraction, two contraction, three contraction, four.

Five contraction, six contraction, seven contraction, sore.

The slippery little body comes quickly. Very quickly. Almost as quickly as our now-dried car, which shot through a couple of reds on the Euston Road in order to arrive just in the nick of time. (Hot Wheels – beat that!)

If the hospital calls to tell you to appear on the scene ... and fast, you do not dilly-dally. Perhaps Dirk might have wished he'd tarried awhile though. When he materialises in the delivery room, his body still reeling from travelling at the speed of light, he is rewarded for his efforts by having the bones in his hands squeezed with astonishing brute force. But he does not carp. This would be the wrong thing to do.

I am like a werewolf, morphing from reasonably normal between contractions into an altogether different beast each time they come. I'm wild-eyed. I grit my teeth violently on the gas and air mouthpiece. I wonder if they ever break? The teeth or the mouthpieces.

With a final howl at the moon I push. Once. Twice. Three times a baby.

Relief.

'It's a little boy Mrs, erm, Mum.'

Little Boy, also occasionally known as 'Testosterone Time-Bomb', is the most sophisticated living species of monkey. It is sometimes said 'Girls are eating Mars, and boys are smearing them in the carpet.' This is fairly accurate, until the age of approximately thirteen, when the girls abstain from Mars, discussing their calorie content instead, whilst the boys continue to smear them in the carpet.

The Little Boy is a species of small monkey that inhabits the islands of Unmade Bed, Muddy Puddle and Tangle of Smelly Socks in Central Scuffsland. A member of the ape family, the Little Boy is the largest semi-civilised species of monkey, growing to an average height of 1 metre 9, occasionally surging to 1 metre 10 when there's a fairground ride height restriction to be reckoned with.

This great length is attributed to eating large quantities of sausages with plenty of ketchup on the side, although it must absolutely not touch the peas or the carrots at any time. As a result of their great size, these monkeys are apex Baked Beanz consumers, dominating the ecosystems in which they live with their frequent and largely repugnant farting competitions.

They prefer damp and mucky terrain, typically galumphing their way through puddles whilst sporting their freshly polished 'good' shoes. Autumn leaves hiding perfidious dog poo are also good. Little Boy usually avoids both of these, however, when wearing his shiny Wellington boots.

As ectotherms, they are most active in the day, although they do exhibit some nocturnal activity, usually when there is a pillow fight in the offing or whisperings of a midnight feast. These occur more often than not when Mummy, also occasionally known as 'Worn-Out Woman', has had a bad day.

Little Boys can be solitary and often quite miffed when banished to the naughty step, coming together only to eat, burp and snigger. They are capable of running rapidly in brief sprints (up to twenty kilometres per hour) when the ice-cream van tinkles 'Greensleeves', are excellent swimmers (though dive-bombing is better), and pee most proficiently against trees or into flowerpots, even when there is a conventional loo within reach.

For shelter, Little Boys make dens from the sofa or with duvets in the bottom bunk. Typically, they run excitably around the house naked before bath time and have a habit of mislaying their dressing gown and slippers when they get out. This makes them poor, in the early evenings, at conserving body heat.

Fortunately, that is where Mummy comes in handy, providing a warm lap, a hug and a mug of hot milk before bedtime. Unless Little Boy has drawn on the wall or his younger sibling again in which case it's straight to bed with no cuddles.

Apgar completed, they envelop Billy in a white towel and hand him over to us. He is 5 lb 11 oz, small but perfectly formed. He will need looking after but mercifully he seems OK.

I'm still a bit in shock at the speed of events. I take my baby in my arms and look down. I see that, indeed, it is a baby boy. No denying that one. Another boy is good, I think. A football buddy. An echo for Tarzan games in our back-garden jungle. A partner in crime for tongue-rolling experiments and turning eyelids inside out. Jack will be made up. And me? I have the excuse to lobby for another one. My baby is less than five minutes old, I'm reeling from a violent labour and I'm already planning the next.

I shiver slightly, pause and then commence babbling. I apologise for my screaming banshee act, I look for reassurance that my bowels didn't let me down in a crisis and I begin manically thanking everyone for their performance, like an emotional and rambling Oscar-clutching Gwynnie. Sadly I haven't managed to slip into a pale pink Ralph Lauren dress for the occasion, and I don't at this moment, or ever, in fact, look as good as her under the spotlight. Still, at least I'm not going to try to breastfeed an apple, I suppose.

Kindly, nobody tells me to snap out of it. Instead, while Dirk disappears with the baby for precautionary neo-natal checks, I gently peter out. I savour the proffered hot sweet tea and toast whilst trying, a bit calmer now, to take it all in.

Jack, at eighteen months little more than a baby himself, is overjoyed at the arrival of his new brother. He is all over the Moses basket with strokes, brotherly cooing and big sloppy kisses. It is love at first sight. Billy, with barely opened eyes and a deep frown furrowing his diminutive brow, is reserving judgement.

Jack loves his new brother so much he wants to play with him all the time. He pushes Billy in the battery-operated baby swing, even stronger when the crying increases in case that makes it better. He points out car pictures to him in his favourite board book. He pushes his beloved Bertie Bus into the folds of Billy's sheets. He seems smitten with his new little playmate.

I in turn gaze lovingly at the pair of them. Billy is Little. Jack is Large. They make a comedy duo; Jack seems gargantuan next to his wee slip of a tiny sidekick. His thighs, his head and his bottom seem massive. He also looks like Einstein on a bad hair day. I make a mental note to book him in for a cut. Because, in his new capacity as 'big brother' and all round brick, he's worth it.

Jack is oblivious to our hilarity at the sight of them side by side. He moons over his bestest new playmate in the world and sighs. If it was the right time of year, I have no doubt he would pick a fresh daisy and contentedly picked off all the petals one by one. 'He loves me, he loves me not, he loves me, he loves me not ...'

He would of course engineer a grand 'he loves me' finale to finish on. Not sure what Scarlett, his hitherto first and only love, might make of this fickle behaviour, but it's hard to play by the gentlemanly rules when you're small and thoroughly besotted.

Jack has cheerfully accepted that now he will need to share his toys, the bath and his changing mat. He has cheerfully accepted the usurping of his place in the pushchair, taken to the new buggy board like Avril Lavigne's rad sk8ter boy dude, and cheerfully accepted the need to share Mummy and Daddy with all the grace of a thoroughly good egg.

I am delighted. He seems to have accepted Billy in spite of any fears I may have harboured of sibling jealousy or rejection. There is never any mention on his part of sending the baby back to the shop. But the baby, however, is very nearly taken back of its own accord.

Jack and Billy went up the hill to fetch a pail of water
Jack fell down, bounced back like a clown and Billy came
    tumbling after

Up Jack got, wiped off the snot, picked up the fallen
    daisies
Recovered his head, did drawing instead, with crayons
    and sugar paper.

Only Billy didn't pick himself up from the tumble.

The Whittington Hospital. Early March. I'm back in a boxy
hospital room where it's quiet, cut off from the hubbub in the
corridor outside. The heating's belting out a clammy fug of
heat. It's just me and little Billy kicking contentedly in the
clinical cot.

Dirk's taken Jack back home and will bring me an overnight
bag later. We'd come into the hospital earlier to get Billy
checked over. Something wasn't right. Dirk had gone out with
Jack, leaving me time to rest a little. Billy was in on the plot,
allowing me to take it easy for a bit while he dozed in his Moses
basket. He was, I thought gleefully, still in sleepy mode. They do
that at first, babies, sleep a lot. I know, I've already had one. It's
only once they've lulled you into a false sense of security that
something turns and they start baying for milk, burps and
ablutions from dusk until dawn. But not Billy. Not yet. Lucky
me, I thought as I lolled on the sofa, better make the most of it
while I can.

I put it down to him being an early bird. He was now two
weeks, that's thirty-seven weeks in gestation terms. Should've
still been inside. He was probably just lying back pondering
what it was to be Aquarian and not a Pisces-Arian cusp case
which would've been altogether different, or chuckling
appreciatively at landing a birthday next to Valentine's Day; it'll
do wonders for his future street cred when the morning post

arrives. Actually, he was most likely just in a daze because he was knackered. It's tiring being regularly up in the wee small hours. After all, I should know.

Gosh, he was very quiet though. I roused myself from the sofa to check on him: cup a hand around his cheek, check he was warm at the neck under his vest, reassure myself he was OK. But he wasn't. To my horror, he seemed odd. He was still, and a strange colour. I panicked. I was alone, what could I do? I reached for my book: *What to Expect* ... when the unexpected happened.

Premature and new babies, I learned, often have difficulties with regulating their circulation. Don't worry about purplish mottling — it's just a sign of your baby's immature circulation. I looked back into the cot, still a bit shaken, and was relieved to see he was open-eyed, stirring and a normal-looking colour once again. Silly me. Perhaps I had imagined it? I caressed him again. Now he seemed fine. Nothing to worry about, then. And anyway, I'm a second-time mum now. Much more laid back this time. Silly me.

Except a little later, it happened again. And again, for longer this time. Dad popping in for a flying visit, agreed that something was not quite right. Dirk, returning from his well-meaning absence, bundled us all in the car, roared up the Holloway Road and into A&E quick as a flash. We were seen instantly. If ever you want to avoid a lengthy A&E wait, just claim to be under two and you'll be seen then and there. Though to be fair, the triage nurse might soon smell a rat when she notices you're out of short trousers.

I'd felt a bit daft. He now looked right as rain. Nothing to worry about at all. Probably wasting everyone's time. But the doctor took it seriously and embarked on a series of tests. These included taking a urine sample, which was enough to make a grown-man wince. OK, so there was no hair involved, but did they really need to *sellotape* the bag around his tender bits?

Everything had seemed very measured. Jack was playing delightedly with the hospital toys in the background. I had to repeat what had happened before a medical student and felt, again, as though I was here on false pretences. They were probably checking my story to see if it tallied with the earlier version.

I was fairly sure they'd send us home soon, tail between legs. 'It's always best to check if in doubt, but anyone can plainly see this baby is pink as the day he was born. Oh, OK, so he was yellow then? Well, he's not yellow now. Come on, then, be off with you this instant!'

Only that's not what happened. This is what did:

'Right then, we're having a cot made ready for him on Ifor Ward. I'm afraid you won't be going home tonight.'

'Oh?' I stuttered. 'I thought he seems fine now?'

'He may *seem* fine. But with what you've told us earlier, we'll be keeping him in for obs. Better safe than sorry eh?'

Rules for Playing Safe on the Ward

Mothers of Paediatric In-Patients must follow these rules when staying on our ward:

- You may walk up the ward corridor for jugs of water, borrowing the electric breast pump and/or going to the toilet when you can't put it off any longer. Running is not allowed.
- Fighting is not permitted anywhere, any time. Even if the consultant takes *for ever* to show up for the ward round, and then has the cheek to tell you stuff you don't want to hear – perhaps in front of a crowd of students to add insult to injury – lay off him or her, or else.
- Shoes stay off feet. You must wear slippers from now until

discharge. It will either make you feel at home and/or as though you're starting to feel ill youself.

- Only nurses are allowed to move or rearrange equipment. Other than IV drips which are constantly tripping. You may wish to deactivate the alarm before your ears go doo-lally, but you must summon a nurse immediately after, taking care not to trigger the emergency call button which will result in an all-out staff sprint to your bedside followed by an all-out staff grump for being a time-waster.
- The grotty patient kitchen where you can make yourself a cuppa is to be shared by *everyone*.
- When interacting with the nurses use kind words. This means everyone is included. No one should make fun of or bully the nurses. Trust me, you don't want a nurse to nurse a grudge.

And so here I am, making us both cosy in another sterile hospital room. Billy's in another Perspex cot, wrapped in another candlewick blanket. It is fleshy pink this time, the colour of old-fashioned elastoplasts.

A senior nurse comes in clutching a clipboard. She's petite and pretty with a ready smile and an earthy voice. She picks up Billy's small hand and strokes his fingers. I take it as affection and warm to her immediately. But then she rubs her thumb across his fingernails with increased urgency and frowns.

'Are they always like this?'

I look down at his hands. I see ten tiny digits, which are adorable and seem, to me, as hands should be. Are they always like this? I think so. But then again, I haven't gazed indulgently at him for hours on end like my firstborn. It's been busier this time. I've admired of course. But I don't know. I don't *know* if his hands are any different.

I start to burble apologetically, kicking myself for not being better. But she's not listening anyway. She hits the button above the bed, an alarm sounds and all chaos breaks out.

> A mummy went to A & E
> To see what's wrong with her Billy
> But all that she could see see see
> Was the bottom of the nurse running swiftly

She flies out of the room pushing the wheeled cot at full tilt. I run forlornly after her. The coffee machine change in my pockets jangles with every step. I feel like I'm in *Casualty* and any moment now the camera will stop running and we can all relax. But it's not like that.

Doctors and nurses come running from all directions. They all head into the room labelled Resuscitation. I follow.

They've got him on the bed. He looks tiny on it, lying on that disposable blue paper they unroll and tear off for each patient. I'm silently praying he's not disposable too. Not going to be torn off and thrown in the bin.

Please God. He's only just arrived. Please don't take him from me already.

They're fanning oxygen over his face. He's blue. I'm standing in the corner of the room, numb. A kindly nurse encircles my shoulders. He's turning pinkish again. He's breathing.

'It's going to be OK,' she whispers.

'Is it moving?'

'Has it lost another leg?'

A worn fish tank that has seen better days is centre of attention on the middle of our kitchen table. Three small heads are crowding around, breathing condensation onto the jaded Perspex their noses are so close.

We have been charged with looking after a small colony of stick insects for a week in the holidays while our opposite neighbour is away. She herself is caring for them for her son who is involved with an educational ecology centre that has closed over the summer now that school's out.

The beleaguered stick insects have been passed from pillar to post. One has only two legs left. It is either very careless or has been picked up far too many times by heavy-handed junior botanists.

'There's the other one. I can see it, I can see it!'

'Is that its poo or eggs?'

We have a lot to learn.

There's a name for it, a blue episode. Forgetting to breathe. Having a not-at-all funny turn. 'Apnoea'. Sounds like a hardy perennial that'd light up your borders or look good in a part-shaded patio container (well mulched).

I like blue. I wear a lot of it. The curtains and cushions in my house seem to be ninety per cent blue. I like that stuff that you put in the back of the loo that makes the water turn all blue when you flush. Kind of makes the whole event much more exciting. Blue is the colour of forget-me-nots, infinity and proper cheese and onion crisps. (Second-rate cheese and onion crisps are yellow and green.)

I love bluebells in our garden in spring. They're beautiful but they're also nobody's fool. They fill the garden with a froth of pretty blue, but behind the front they're a bunch of toughies. They self-seed and spread almost imperceptibly. They outnumber and outlast the paltry tulips. And they stick their tongues out and waggle their fingers in the faces of the bully-boy bad guys, saying 'pah' to the marauding squirrels and munch-hungry snails who usually lord it round here. For that I love them all the more.

But there are places, however, where I do not love blue. On football shirts for starters, being loyal to my patch. Flashing on ambulances. In moods. On the edges of your loaf just when you'd fancied some toast. In humour, the toilet variety being more my kind of level these days.

And I do not like blue on my child's fingertips and lips. It is not a good look.

Billy had drifted in and out of a couple of worrying apnoea episodes that night. I'd silently watched, feeling impotent and kicking myself for not coming in sooner. Maybe this could've been avoided if I'd trusted my initial instincts? Maybe I should've come in the first time I saw something?

Dirk came back with an overnight bag slung over his shoulder having left Jack with a neighbour. He was mildly perplexed when he found the room where he'd left us empty. The worst was now over though. He took over sentry role by the well-tended resus bed while I was led to a small room and offered tea and toast. A weird throwback to the post-labour feast I'd laid into a couple of weeks previously. I couldn't face the toast. I wept instead.

Jack returns triumphant, having snipped some twigs from the privet hedge out front. Billy is carefully extracting the old, wilted ones, trying to avoid bringing a stick insect or just one of his dismembered legs aloft at the same time. He fumbles and drops some leaves on the tabletop. Sid shrinks instinctively, maintaining a safe distance, watching in utter awe of proceedings.

'Mummy, can *we* get some? I really like them!'

'Well, we could but *you* would be the ones who'd have to care for them. *You* would have to change the leaves and give them fresh water. Regularly. And clean out the poo.'

'Can we then?'

'And not expect Mummy to do it when you get bored.'

'Course not.'

'No. Never.'

'Never!'

'*I'd* want them to have babies! That'd be *so* cool.'

'Yeah, cute little baby ones.'

One could, I'm sure, find many ways to describe the humble stick insect. I'm not sure 'cute' would be one of them.

'Let's just see how keen you are at the end of the week, shall we?'

By the end of the week, I am the one watering our house guests and trying valiantly to resist the urge to gloat 'I told you so.' I am quite pleased when we return the tank from where it came. With all delivered stick insects still hale and hearty, and boasting the same number of limbs that they arrived with.

No babies that I noticed though.

Not yet knowing what was wrong, they'd zapped him with antibiotics and pulled him back from the brink. They were still unsure what had prompted the gremlins to steal up from behind and snatch away Billy's natural instinct to breathe. And they were unsure of what the long-term developmental consequences might be. But at least he was out of critical danger.

I spent the twilight hours quietly feeding him, going over and over my silent apologies. I would trade anything to have him well. I would give my right arm. I was sorry I hadn't come sooner. I was desperately sorry I was thinking of *other* babies within minutes of his birth. I didn't want other babies. I wanted this one. To take care of, to nurture and to see grow into a healthy and happy, normal boy. I was so, so sorry.

• • •

A few nights later, we are still in the Whittington. Billy's tiny hand has a cannula lodged in and he's strung up to a drip metering out I/V antibiotics. We're out of danger. He's doing well. He's breathing for himself normally, and I'm breathing easier too. But he'd worried me for a bit then.

I can hear the foxes calling out in Waterlow Park just beyond the windows. It's a weird sort of shrieking which seems at odds with the debonair look of the fox who you'd somehow imagine would speak with a devilishly deep-voiced caddish swagger.

I think of Scamp who I've still got somewhere at home. I'll have to pull him out of retirement, dust him off and give him to Billy.

The shrieking in my own head has calmed a bit now. I've had a lot of time to think.

Some weeks later. We're in Cambridge visiting my parents. I'm in the kitchen with Mum. She's at the worktop chopping parsley. She's holding the knife with both hands, one at each end of the blade. There's a rhythmic drumming as the green fronds are quickly and effectively pulverised. I've never been able to do it like that.

I'm sitting at the kitchen table feeding Billy. Dad and Dirk have taken Jack out to the swings.

'Mum. What did you hope for in your children?'

She puts the knife down and looks at me quizzically.

'Are you getting philosophical, then, in your old age?'

'No, I'm just interested, that's all.'

'What did I hope for? Oooh, everything and anything. You just want the best for your children, don't you?'

'Like what?'

'You want for things to turn out OK. You want that they don't get hurt. You want them to be happy.'

I look down at the still-fragile little boy in my arms. He's had needles stuck in his hands, his feet and his head as they tried to find a big enough blood-yielding vein, he's had a lumbar puncture and he's had a transparent plastic bag sellotaped to his willy.

When the tests finally came back, it turned out it was meningitis. He is still frail-looking, a little pale and undersized. We don't yet know what the long-term consequences might be. But he's still with us.

This little fella had us all worried then for a bit. But now I've been through it with him, I'm bowled away by the bond I've developed with this knocked-about little lad. And I want him to be with us now for the innings. I know above all that he is undeniably part of the family now, that it is right for Jack to have a sibling with whom to share our affections. I also no longer give a toss about whether his clothes are pink or blue. I just want his skin to remain firmly in the pink camp, thank you very much.

Things are still, by the skin of their teeth, OK. And me? Yes, I'm still hurting a bit in aftershock, but I am without a doubt happy.

Mum comes over and puts her arm around my shoulders. We look down at my younger son. I can smell the comforting homely smell of parsley on her fingers.

Chapter 11

Some of us take on having a second baby hot on the heels of the first for a variety of reasons. We embrace the 'two under two' madness because we want to avoid going out again to make ends meet, grab a chance to immerse ourselves in the work we really enjoy and/or create a new and special, though sometimes chaotic project that we can look back on in our dotage and say 'What the chuffing heck did we do that for then?' Or sometimes we just have an 'accident' and run with it.

No matter the reason for opting for this approach, juggling more than one under-two is guaranteed to be a crash course in time management, solutions-finding and moderation of jangled nerves.

How to do it, then? How do you juggle more than one under-two?

Managing Multiple Under-Twos at Once: Tips to Stay on Top!

i) *Remember who's in charge.* You are the mummy. Hold your head high. Even when old ladies tut you for daring to emerge in daylight and bring your double buggy into Londis. Remember, even they were small once. And besides, double buggy wheels do tend to ram into the ankles of busybodies, I find.

ii) *Create and use effective time-management tools.* A Parisian scenes calendar on the fridge may look pretty, but it's no use to anyone if you don't write in the immunisations appointment, the play date with George and your physio consultation for back pain treatment (hoiking two small people around day in, day out, can be heavy work). Also, remember to ensure that you can see it at all times. You will never get to where you need to be on time if the schedule is covered with alphabet magnets, party invites and sugar-paper masterpieces.

iii) *Prioritise.* When a crisis comes up with baby A while you're supposed to be taking care of something for baby B, you will have to choose between your needy babies. The best you can do is defer to age. Give precedence to the child who is bigger and louder. The younger one will not remember lying abandoned, screaming with hunger/wind/ indignation in its cot while you tend to the bloodied knee of the older one. Unfair I know. That's life, I'm afraid, kiddo.

iv) *Find a rhythm and set a schedule to fit around it.* Don't expect to leave the house before lunchtime. Don't expect to go out anywhere for lunch anyway. Go nowhere you can't manage without a double buggy. (Most places then.)

v) *Plan the work and then work the plan.* No day with two under-twos will go one hundred per cent as planned. An effective mummy must be able to overcome one child's desire to get up close and personal with the 3-in-1 toilet rim freshener whilst changing the nappy of the other on a raised surface. Useful assets in situations like these are having eyes in the back of your head and three pairs of hands. One set at least should be extendable.

vi) *Develop your decision-making skills.* You will need to address challenges like how to shift two small children from the car parked on the road outside your house and get the shopping in without mishap and/or being charged for child neglect. This set-up can be further complicated if you're foolhardy enough to have a dog, in which case you regularly have to figure out the 'fox, two chickens, river and one boat' conundrum. Paying for your petrol at the petrol station can also be a toughie.

vii) *Keep an eye on the big picture concepts.* Pretty much all children will learn to walk and read some time. But if you don't help them along, you'll be forever beating yourself up if they're behind their contemporaries. It will be useful, therefore, to learn fairly early on how to breastfeed whilst coaching your other child through Dr Seuss's ABC on your other knee. Cooking tea at the same time would be a bonus.

viii) *Focus on what is important.* Face it. You are outnumbered, but you have two hands. One for each child. You will manage.

I am wearing a white coat, yellow plastic goggles and a whacky Technicolor tie. I have a gawkish grin and my hair is quite mad. Today, boys and girls, I am Charlotte MixItUpAndPourMan, chemistry teacher extraordinaire. 'Good morning boys and girls. I hope everyone is sitting comfortably. Today's lesson should be rather an exciting one.'

'As you know, children, I love experimenting. I will try anything once.'

(Giggles and shuffling amongst the crowd.)

'And so, for our first experiment, let's produce a small child in a puff of green smoke.'

BANG!

Enter, Jack.

(Gasps. Applause.)

What I did

- I took two large fairly average pots, one slightly bigger than the other.
- From the bigger pot I took two teaspoons of gunk, added a couple of small drops of green food colouring for effect, and poured them into the smaller pot. (That was the fun bit.)
- In the smaller pot I mixed in a gallon of peppermint tea and a packet of Maltesers.
- Then I sat back on a comfy chair and waited a bit. (This part of the experiment can often take some time.)
- Now for another fun bit. I picked someone I'd never met before to reach into the small pot and grab the gooey ball inside. How's that for audience participation?
- I found an old but clean hankie and wrapped the blob in it.

REMARKS

Everything is made from tiny particles called molecules. What came out of the pot was a rather super polymer (that's a lot of molecules joined together). I've called it a blob, but you all now the resulting polymer as ... you've guessed it, our very own Jack!

(More applause.)

'Good, isn't it?'

Jack of course didn't stick to being a small ball of goo. He soon grew and he grew into the most agreeable little fellow you can imagine. He is affectionate. He gives a great cuddle. He thinks he will marry Scarlett. He can recite all the baddies in *Dr Who* with his eyes tight shut. He is mad for all playground trends. He sings, a lot. He is blond and blue-eyed and there's an angry birthmark behind his ear. This is the angriest bit about him. He is not especially tall, but not especially small. In my eyes he is perfect. He is, and will forever be, my firstborn and I love him.

'What do you think kids; have we got time for another?'

A chorus of 'yay!'s, 'all right's and 'if you must's.

'Great! I knew you'd see it my way. And so, for our second experiment, let's produce another small child. We can dispense with the green smoke if you like.'

FIZZ!

Enter, Billy.

Intakes of breath. Clapping.

'Not bad, huh?'

What I did

- I took the same two fairly average pots, one still slightly bigger than the other.
- From the bigger pot I took more gunk, held on the food colouring this time because the idea is frankly a bit odd, and poured it into the smaller pot. (That was still pretty fun, actually.)
- Then I took a bicycle pump, some sticky tape and a cork and I pumped up the smaller pot till it got really big. (This part of the experiment can once again require some patience.)
- When I judged it was big enough – you'll know this just by 'feel', though sometimes everything might be ready to pop sooner than you'd think – I stood back, pumped a bit more at arm's length and observed the explosive launch.

HORRIBLE MESS WARNING!

Please note this part of the experiment can get soggy. Make sure you don't stand too close.

- The pressure inside the pot has been built up to such an extent that eventually it has nowhere else to go but out.
- This was when ... ta da ... Billy cannonballed out.

'Wow!'

Billy is also blond with big blue eyes. His best buddy in all the world is Luka, brother of Scarlett. I don't *think* he intends to marry him, but you never know. Billy is happy to sidle up to family, friends and strangers alike and engage them in earnest conversation. He chuckles infectiously when he's pulling a new stunt or trick. He loves to clown around under a blanket playing the 'I am invisible' game, whizz grinningly down the hill on his bike and enthusiastically point out random instances of the letter 'B' on number plates, shop signs and passing vans. Especially ice-cream vans. He is obsessed by robbers and death and poo. He loves making biscuits and licking out the bowl. He gives sloppy kisses, eats 'white' yoghurts dropping globules down his top and is a secret seedless-grape sneaker. He plays trains, builds Lego and dresses up in all manner of outlandish polyester costumes.

We never forget what a gift he is to still have and to hold. He is a complex, intriguing character, and I utterly adore him.

'Well, kids, it's nearly the end of the period. We might just have time to fit in another. Risk getting another one in under the wire before the bell goes eh?'

Grumbles and sucking of teeth.

'Oh, go on. Don't be so boring. Life's never fun unless you take a few risks! More! More! We want more!'

'Yeah, OK then, Miss. But be quick about it.'

(Titters in the back row.)

'Ooh, I do love it when you're keen. Let's see. Ah yes. I *had* been getting on top of things, Managing, in a manner of speaking. One hand for each child when the Lab Technician's away. Bit boring eh? Bit too easy?'

'Whatever you say, Miss.'

'Here we go then. Let's take some vinegar, Diet Coke and Potassium PerMoermanate $DCbO_{y3}$, bung them all together in a centrifuge, switch on and see what happens shall we?'

FLASH!

'Ah yes, now we're talking. Let the real fun and games begin.'

(Gulps.)

* * *

I am thirty-six weeks. I'm in bed. It is late. I roll over and then, downstairs, I suddenly burst like a water bomb. I leap from the covers, sprightlier than I have been for weeks, nay years and gush all over the floor.

'What the ...?'

'Looks like my waters have gone,' I say, illustrating the point with another thorough floor dousing. 'Here we go again ...' OK, so I'm speeding things up here, but you know that's the lot of the third child. It's squeezed into the schedule, dealt with and then we're off onto something new.

I sit on the toilet, expertly allowing the remaining fluid to drain off into the sewers instead of over the upholstery of our car.

The midwives want us in again after last time. They never knew for sure, but Billy's infant meningitis may have been caused by my having Strep B (or Group B Streptococcus if we're being formal. Sounds like a dinosaur only you can't spot this one coming through the undergrowth). It may have also been because of the length of time between my waters breaking and delivery, which allowed an infection to creep in. Or it could have been just one of those unlucky things. Bit of bad luck. Either way, we're not taking any risks.

It is after hours. The boys have long been tucked up in bed. Nick our neighbour comes around and sleeps on the sofa while we head off to our old friend the Elizabeth Garrett Anderson.

I am seen quickly. I'm allocated a bed. I'm told it's a waiting game. I am getting a sense of déjà vu.

'They usually come within twenty-four hours of the waters breaking,' says one of the night nurses.

I know, I think, as I assess my proximity to the stairs, wondering how many times I'll trudge up and down them in a bid to get things moving. Or indeed how close we are to the lifts and whether I'm going to be doing another *Supermarket Sweep*-style trolley dash to get in and out of them.

'Just a flying visit, Chaz,' says Dad, taking off his suit jacket and hanging it on the back of a chair.

Dad works in London and occasionally, for a lunchtime treat, tubes up to Arsenal.

'Grandpa, Grandpa. Let's play snap.'

He switches off from the hubbub, the demands of work and that dying breed – a chain-smoking colleague at his desk – by zipping in for a game of cards, a tomato sandwich and the chance to bond with his grandsons.

He sits patiently at the kitchen table. The boys crane expectantly over the wipe-clean vinyl cloth decorated with multicoloured circles and strawberries. Their legs are folded underneath them like contortionists'. They are ready at any second to spring into orbit with the pent-up excitement of it all.

In front of them is a set of large Postman Pat cards, face down in two piles. Jack, by dint of being the eldest, has taken centre stage opposite his grandpa who *may* have the benefit of approximately sixty years on his side but seems to be remarkably slow about calling Snap.

On the exaggerated nod, they both turn over the top card. Dad does a slow-motion stagey flip while Jack nimbly flicks his over without a moment to lose. He is biting his nails in nervous anticipation.

'Will it be ...? Is it ...? Oh, no! Postman Pat and Mrs Goggins. Not this time.'

They turn the next cards over. This time there are two Ted Glens. Everyone has seen them, me and Dad, the builders over the back, all seven astronauts floating around the International Space Station.

'SNAP!' calls Jack eventually in triumph, soon echoed by a sibling eager to share in the glory.

'Oh, you got me there, you rascal. Quick off the mark this one, eh Chaz?'

'Lightning-quick, Grandpa.'

Pelmanism had been my game of choice at that age. I would play it for hours if I could. Dad was the stooge then too.

It's the same principle as Snap. You're looking for pairs. There's comfort in matching things. Recognising the familiar.

I've given birth twice now. Both experiences were poles apart. I wonder if third time round will pan out like one that I've already got under my belt, or if I'm going to go down a completely new route.

So far so like birth number two. My waters have broken early. I'm waiting around for the action to hot up. And yes, the same hospital curtains are surrounding me with their enveloping yellow pallor. Same old, same old.

But unlike last time when I waited in a solitary side room, I am back on the post-natal ward, biding my time in a room full of women with their already-born babies. What is more, I may well be going back to theatre in the morning if the contractions don't start in the interim. Nobody wants to leave it too long and risk a repeat of last time's infection or whatever it was that hexed us.

So maybe we'll wind up like birth number one again then? I'm hoping not to be honest. Having tried both methods, I can definitely say that Mother Nature has it all sewn up so to speak. To be opened like a trapdoor, rifled through and stitched back together was the quieter but in my opinion the much less preferable way of delivering a baby. I want another VBAC. (That's Vaginal Birth after Caesarean to remove any doubt for those wondering if I want a new hoover attachment.) Maybe a trifle slower than last time, but that's the method I'd prefer.

Of course the method was great but the after-events were pants.

If I could pick and choose then, my ideal would be to turn over the card that looked like birth number two. But I'd also want to pick the one that looked like the ensuing good health of baby number one.

I wonder what I'll actually get dealt then.

It is morning now and I am counting my blessings. The consultant who came on listened to my pleas to avoid surgery if we could. So instead of going straight into theatre at nine, I'm being allowed until teatime to see if, with the help of an induction drip, I can huff and puff and win this showdown.

I am lucky, I'm of the era where there's choice. Choice to take a pill to stop you falling pregnant if you wish. Choice to abort a baby if the arrangement doesn't suit. And choice – although this is one you sometimes *most* have to fight for – to try and push a baby out through the undercarriage rather than ejecting it through the sunroof if humanly possible.

And so here I am, all tubed and wired up, waiting to find out if I can beat the deadline. This time I've got a midwife permanently in attendance. I'm on the drip to speed up labour. I'm being monitored for foetal anxiety and stress on my C-Section scar. I've been nil-by-mouth since dawn and am back in a gown and TED stockings in case we need to rush into theatre. I watch the slow progression of the clock hands. The pace of events at least couldn't be more different from my last labour if it tried.

There's a window open. I remember being overwhelmingly hot last time. This time, it is icy instead. The midwife starts to sniffle. We close the window and she smiles, pulling out a Kleenex. I shift on the bed. It would be nice to be able to close a window on my discomfort too, but it's not that simple. I am sitting on the bed, unable to move off it. The small of my back is an ongoing dull ache, but the real action is a way off beginning yet. I just have to sit, wait and watch the teeny contractions on the monitor.

The hands on the wall clock continue to dawdle around at snail pace. It's the *Countdown* clock on marijuana, the chilled-out, why hurry, pole-opposite to speed. I count the revolutions on the clock. Slowly. A painfully sluggish stopwatch to theatre.

Unless of course baby beats the clock.

'Here's one coming,' says Dirk as he watches the monitor intently.

'Thanks,' I say as I grit my teeth.

I'm still at the stage where I remember my manners.

The clock ticks on.

• • •

When I broke my ankle, I got the ambulance with flashing lights and everything. They took me to Hillingdon Hospital. I waited on a trolley in A&E. Being a little older than two, I had to politely wait my turn.

Dirk was flying to San Francisco at the time, unaware of what was going on. I'd called my parents briefly before being told to switch off my mobile by a fierce-looking nurse. I'd assured them I'd be fine and call them from home in the morning before hanging up.

Some time later I was wheeled into an anteroom. Here, they explained, they would try pushing my ankle back into line with the rest of my leg. I felt nauseous. It soon became clear I wouldn't be going home that night.

They offered me gas and air, which I sucked in with deep, desperate breaths. The room began to pulsate around me. The blurred nurses converged on the bed and my eyes nearly popped out of my head. The procedure was swiftly carried out and done, but I continued to take deep inhalations of the deliciously dizzy-making gas. Every cloud has a silver lining.

Well-practised in the art of inhaling Entonox, I draw in another deep lungful and lie my head back. It's also known as laughing gas, but I can't feel myself about to break into chuckles. I focus on a spot on the ceiling and sing 'Joy to the World' to myself over and over again to take the focus off the pain.

'So last time I stuck to gas and air,' I mumble to the midwife. 'When do I get the chance to upgrade?'

'Let's just wait a while, till the consultant comes in,' she says. 'They said you'd be into theatre if this baby's not here within the hour, so let's not do anything rash.'

An hour? I'm ready to do anything rash as long as the pain goes away. Take me to theatre if you like. Bring me the paperwork, I'd sign on the dotted line for anything right now. Nobody switch on QVC, I might buy something ridiculous.

Times goes on. The clock goes tick tock, the clock goes tick tock, it's time to say: 'No, I can't wait much longer. Can we start talking epidurals, please?'

'Erm, actually, it looks like it's all systems go,' she counters briskly. 'No time for epidurals. Baby will be with us soon.'

'What do you mean, no time?'

'Here comes another one,' chips in Dirk helpfully.

'OK. Hold. Hold. That's right.'

Dirk has spent large chunks of time in foreign climes. He has been to four different continents since the birth of our first child, often two in the same week, and then again the week after. He's worked in Beruit, Dubai and Khartoum. He's been in Bombay, Tanzania and all around the Stans. He's been to Lesotho, Singapore and occasionally to Slough. He's been away, or going through a tunnel, more than you'd care to imagine.

He grips hold of my hand, just like last time. He is here right now and that is where I need him. My eyes are tight closed, but I know he's there. I know because he is talking ten to the dozen in my left ear. It is exactly what I need to help me focus. He is in his stride now, talking me through it just like when I'm trying to parallel park. Only more tense if that is possible.

'You're doing brilliantly. Keep going. You started the manoeuvre well. You've got your rear bumper lined up beautifully. That's right. Hold it there. Hold. Hold. OK, it's all looking safe. But you mustn't push yet. Think reverse. Reverse. Reverse. You're doing just great.'

I'm ready to go now. When will it be time? Let me release the handbreak. I'm desperate to step on the gas, sink my teeth into the Entenox mouthpiece and at last find the biting point.

And then finally they say push. And I push. And I scream and they say,'Don't scream, Charlotte.' (Things have changed since the first time, they now all address me by my first name.) And I think I bloody well will scream if I want to. It helps. Another contraction. I let my lungs go for it hammer and tongs. Though fortunately no actual tongs are required as after one, two, three pushes, out he comes. Our third son.

The Tale of the Three Little Pigs

(Highbury Reading Tree)

Once upon a time, there were Three Little Pigs aged two minutes, twenty-three months, and approximately three and a half. The pigs were small, and so were the age gaps between them. What they lacked in stature, however, they more than made up for in guts. Each Little Pig had vowed to leave their first home, Mummy Pig's gaff, and go out and find their way in the world.

The first Little Pig was a level-headed and considerate chap. He thought that he would leave at a pre-agreed time. He packed up his belongings, waited to be called and then went calmly and sensibly out into the land of Operating Theatre.

Operating Theatre was a nice enough place. It was clean. There were lots of kind people around. And there was music in the background too. The first Little Pig liked Operating Theatre but he was soon chased out by the big bad Jaundice Giant.

Luckily, after a few huffs and puffs from everyone all round, the first Little Piggy was able to outpace the

Jaundice Giant, and he made his way in the world as happy as can be.

TEACHER'S NOTES
Play a game
> Take a straw poll amongst the class and see if they think this was a good or a bad way for the first Little Pig to make his entrance.

OTHER IDEAS
> Ask the children to retell the story in their own words.
> Encourage the children to write a sentence describing how Mummy Pig might be feeling. Reassure them that, though she was knocked a bit sideways for a while, she was soon able to stand on her own four trotters again.

The second Little Pig wanted to get out of the house as fast as his little legs could carry him. He didn't wait around for Mummy's say so, he just shot out like a tube of stamped-on toothpaste.

He arrived much as he meant to go on: fast-paced and furious in a frenzied kind of place called Delivery Room. He didn't stick around there long and quickly hotfooted off to Neo-Natal, another place he didn't rate much, so he scarpered off from there, too, quick sharp. Only to land back, fairly soon afterwards, in Paediatric In-Patients somewhere Entirely Different.

It was a confusing time for our rush-about second Little Pig. Especially when he was set upon by the big bad

Meningitis Monster – scarier but no less alliterative than the first big bad guy.

Luckily, after quite a considerable number of huffs and puffs from everyone all round, the second Little Pig was able to send the Meningitis Monster packing, and he made his way in the world as happy as can be.

TEACHER'S NOTES
Play a game
> Tell the children the 'what's brown and sticky?' joke. Ask them if they found it funny. (Probably not.) Ask the class if they think that Mummy Pig found the second Little Pig's entrance routine funny. (Probably not.)

OTHER IDEAS
> Ask the children to draw a picture of the Meningitis Monster. (Remember to reassure them that the Meningitis Monster is only make-believe. Apart from for the unfortunate few that is.)
> Encourage the children to write a sentence describing how Mummy Pig might be feeling now. Let them know that this time she was admittedly pole-axed for a bit (never a good situation for a pig to find itself in), but that she eventually regained her trotters with time.

Now Little Pig number three, he was a different fellow all over again. He wanted to leave the house another way entirely. He took his time, enjoying the help of the drugs that were pressed onto him, contentedly watching everyone fret a bit waiting for him to make his appearance.

Eventually, just before the final whistle was blown, the third Little Pig put everyone out of their suspense, stormed into play and performed the winning move.

He found himself more at ease in Delivery Room than Little Pig two had, and stuck around for a while. And though he was a little boy pig, Mummy Pig was quite delighted, this being the last Little Pig that she was ever going to send out into the world. (Probably.)

Much to Mummy Pig's relief, the third Little Pig looked hale and hearty. He was bigger than the other two pigs had been. (He was a right little porker at 6lb 6oz.) He was also much darker and had a digit missing from one of his trotters. Hurrah for Little Pig three; he had succeeded in his aim of being different all over again.

Daddy Pig, who has been a bit quiet in this story so far, wondered if Postman Pig was dark-haired and four-toed, but Mummy Pig knew this was not the case. (Postman Pig was ginger.)

And so, as the sun set over our happy family of Pigs, everyone heaved a huge sigh of relief. It looked as though they were going to avoid excess huffing and puffing this time round. Everyone was happy. Everyone was healthy.

But would they be so for ever after? That, children, is a very good question.

TEACHER'S NOTES
Play a game
> Mummy Pig had been bricking herself about the sending-out of this Little Pig. Set up a role play. Ask the

children to divide up. Half the class should act out the role of the nonchalant third Little Pig, the rest of the class can have a go at being Mummy Pig. (Remember this is an exercise in imagination. Avoid giving out props. Real bricks might cause trouble.)

OTHER IDEAS
> Ask the children to count the number of digits on everyone's trotters.
> Encourage the children to write a sentence describing how Mummy Pig might be feeling this time round. Reassure them that this time she is all blasé. She shouldn't be though, because one of the monsters is about to strike back with a vengeance.

I hadn't wanted to know the sex of any of my unborn children but there was hardly any mistaking the meat and two veg that shouted out at me during my twenty-week scan with this one. I hadn't asked but I'd kind of known. So I was ready and prepared and that was a good thing. And in any case, right now, I am just overjoyed it is over. My last child (I think). Out. Out and seemingly well.

It seems longer than a mere two years since I had made my whispering promises, bargaining for the health of my son in the still and silent hours at the Whittington Hospital. I said then I didn't want other babies. I just wanted Billy. But things had turned out OK, and we decided to have another. How soon we forget. But here he is; my third little boy wonder. Healthy. Beautiful. How could I be anything other than euphoric?

And I am. I'm buzzing with it. My eyes are practically popping out of my head. I am Kelly Holmes breaking through the winning Olympic tape. I am Sarah Ferguson arriving on her wedding day. I am an average kind of girl wearing Impulse who's been startlingly given flowers by some unknown dishy guy. I am the eye of the tiger. I am on top of the world. I am, for this brief moment in time, Superwoman. I wonder how long it will last.

I now have three children under the age of three and a half, I am still echoing 'Joy to the World' around the back of my head and I feel slightly heady as though someone has just told me I've won the lottery jackpot. Which I suppose I have, in a way. I look over at Dirk with an intoxicated smile and I wonder if I am technically crackers.

In the run-up to the third birth, we had gone to John Lewis in Brent Cross to investigate transportation options. I was a bit wary. I didn't do Brent Cross very often, it seemed to be unlucky.

The last time I'd braved it had been at thirty-five weeks in my second pregnancy. We had gone to pick up a new cot mattress, a cellular blanket and a set of first-size nappies from Mothercare. What I hadn't reckoned for was that this would be my last shopping opportunity before the arrival of our baby. Was it the stress of the Brent Cross car park or fending off the windscreen squeedgy wipers at the lights, or had Billy just been keen to pop out and jump into those nappies without further ado? Whatever the case, it was after the Brent Cross experience that my waters had first begun to trickle prematurely.

And so, still a fair way off term with our third, we'd gingerly returned. I took plenty of deep slow breaths, waddled throughout proceedings at a sensibly even pace and eyed up the sit-in shopmobility vehicles with envy. We'd hustled our two small children into the lift, Dirk hoisted Jack up to press the button and we made our way en masse to the nursery department in John Lewis.

'Hello, there. Can I help you?'

'Yes, I wonder if you can,' I reply. I must look in need of help with my two small children and an obviously expectant tummy. Possibly in the family-planning department. 'I wonder what sort of solutions you could recommend for transporting two toddlers and a baby around?'

'Oh yes, I can see you're going to have your hands full!' (Not heard that line before.) 'Do you drive?' (Ha ha ha.)

'Well, yes, I do drive, but not if I can help it. We can manage the baby and the two year-old with the double buggy, but my three-year-old's a reluctant walker. The last thing I want is extra stress on him when the newborn arrives, so I was just wondering what you suggest?'

'Hmm,' she ponders, eyeing me up and down. 'Well, my honest answer is that nothing suitable really springs to mind. You could try fitting a buggy board to a double pushchair but it's not really recommended.'

'So what do people usually do if they've such a short gap?'

'Madam, people usually *don't* have such a short gap.'

Sid, because that is what we called him, had been given the all clear. He was a bit jaundiced but nothing too concerning so we were sent home. And then we bungee-jumped right back again when his Bilirubin levels soared.

Bilirubin, I discover, is something excreted in bile and its levels are elevated in certain diseases. It is responsible for the yellow colour of bruises, the yellow discolouration in jaundice and, inadvertently, the sallowing of my flesh again when I once more find myself back in a horribly familiar yellow-curtained In-Patients' ward.

I kind of like the term. Bilirubin. It sounds a bit rock and roll. He is not the bassist, though Bili, he is the singer. Not necessarily a boy-band lead. Perhaps someone a bit longer in the tooth. Think Bill Nighy in *Love Actually*. Like him, it's a bit rough, this Bilirubin thing. Definitely not a cutie.

I wonder at the irony of having had three children, two of whom have been nabbed by the Bilirubin beast, but the one who is actually named Billy avoided this one at least.

It's not life-threatening this time, but it's not pretty either. Poor little Sid has his heel pricked again. And again. And then again. Apparently he is mean on yielding blood. I'd be pretty mean to someone repetitively pricking the sole of my already-sore foot, so I am with him on this count.

He is readmitted and whisked beneath an ultraviolet light with a 'biliblanket' under his bottom. It is tempting to think we are on holiday as he lies there with a pair of shades over his eyes and teeny tiny premie nappies rolled up to posing pouch proportions for maximum skin-exposure to the rays. I lie on the bed next to him, at rest from the usual demands of my other boys and read. What is it with hospital beds and my capacity to catch up on my reading matter? I get through *The Da Vinci Code*, *Rory and Ita* and *The Time Traveller's Wife*.

I drift through the languorous mists of hospital time where the clock hands dawdle and your blood pumps sluggishly through your veins. I set my alarm to wake up and feed at regular intervals through the night.

Sid improves slightly, develops an umbilical infection and then dips. Bilirubin is stage-diving again. After several nights I go home when Sid is discharged. I go back when he is readmitted as Bili again hits rock bottom. I feel like the Time Traveller's Forgotten Ex, stuck in an ever-repeating time warp.

Chapter 12

Sometimes I lurch through the days feeling a bit like one of those faces I used to make with Mum when I was small. It would either be from a brown paper bag or a wooden spoon. If it was the wooden spoon version, we might have gone deluxe and sellotaped knitting-wool hair on the top. On one side was a happy face, all dimples and curls and a big toothy grin. On the reverse side was a wildly grumpy version of the same, usually with freckles, heavily pencilled frown lines and an exaggerated pout. This side would probably have been more fun to draw. I would happily spend an entire afternoon twisting round between happy face and grumpster. Round and round and round until Paper Bag Girl got dizzy.

Some days, I am the happy version. Sometimes I am not. Sometimes I am so giddy I wonder if the real version of me got lost somewhere along the way.

A Life in the Day: Charlotte Moerman

The full-time mum, 33, lives with her husband – when he cares to drop by – the international gadabout Dirk Moerman, their sons, Jack (3½), Billy (2), Sid (1 month), and an assortment of plastic tat in Highbury, North London

If Sid hasn't woken me at dawn, Jack hops into the bed for a little love before the day starts at 6.30 a.m. Order of feeding is Sid, who's going for it hammer and tongs at any given opportunity right now. Then Jack and Billy, and then me, if I'm lucky. Dirk is probably being fed dinner somewhere at 35,000 feet. I sometimes grab a cup of tea, and on a good day I'll manage a shower too. Those are few and far between at the moment though, so more often than not, it's straight up to the bedroom for a quick change into my work gear.

I'd like to say that I wear smart casuals, mostly from Gap, plus a couple of smartish dresses for occasions. I'm sure I used to, but they all seem to have mysteriously vanished from my wardrobe. These days, I tend to pull on the same old thing; combats and camouflage. Not that I'm into excess pockets or brown and green splodges, but I am ready at all times to do battle and I have a habit of blending into the background.

An observer might sometimes have trouble locating me. Like Wally in those *Where's Wally?* books. You'd think you'd have no problems picking him out in a crowd in that get-up of his. Hiking boots and a woolly hat. In a swimming pool. But no, he is so surrounded by rubber rings, armbands, floats and other paraphernalia, plus a cornucopia of semi-naked patrons utterly ignoring the signs asking them to kindly refrain from running, bombing, petting, etc, that he just sort of melts into the background.

Once a week a woman comes with a hoover and clears a path through the toys. We like to keep them happy, in well-spaced piles all around the house. Wouldn't be right to overcrowd them. Our favourites are Pat, Bob, Sam, a plastic horse called 'horse' and a great big noisy red rocket.

Lunch for me is just a sandwich. Usually at around half three, once I've met the varying culinary demands of my choosy young charges. I don't pine for work because I know I'll always have a relationship with it. I frequently look up former colleagues on Facebook.

Depending how much exercise they've had, and the calories they've burnt, the boys have a bit of a mad hour around bath time. Those that can walk canter up and down the stairs naked, while I slump defeated on a fold-out chair next to the running taps. I usually have to ask several times for them to stop careering about and get into the bath. Sometimes, it's as though they don't see or hear me at all, the buggers.

Then it's a matter of processing them for the night. Bedtime for the bigger boys is 7 p.m., with stories. I say bigger, but it's all relative of course. We love *Duffy Driver* and the *Little Red Train*. (Toot toot!)

By 9 p.m. I'm knackered, but with a new baby it's anyone's guess when I'll get my kip in. I go out like a light when I can though. Shortly after wondering if Dirk is sleeping, awake or having his breakfast up above the clouds somewhere.

I sit for a moment, staring blankly out the window. I am barely conscious of the white noise all around. I am used to it; I now have fully comprehensive surround-sound as a backdrop to my life. It all came free as part of the package, and you can't say that about many things these days.

Perhaps I should have stopped to think about what I was signing up for before delving in. But no, here I am. Perhaps only now for the first time considering the consequences of our actions. I have three under three and a half. I have two in nappies. I have a headache a lot of the time. I sometimes think I might have woken up in the midst of a Dolby technology cinematic experience. The audience are sitting back in their seats, 3D glasses on, bracing themselves for action. The opening credits roll:

> A long time ago,
> in a galaxy far, far away...
> MA's FLOORED

The audience gasps as a Rebel Toddler, striking from a hidden behind-the-sofa cushion den, does battle against the evil Fraternal Empire. They wonder at the shadowy Far-Off Vader figure. And they pity the seemingly fragile Ma. By rights she should be restoring peace and harmony to the galaxy, but first she needs to find time to double-doughnut her hair. Or even just brushing it might be nice.

I've gazed out the window long enough. Sid needs feeding, the bigger boys need diverting, it is time to take control. I flick on the CD for *Room on the Broom*, hoping that the bigger boys can amuse themselves by acting out the story while I feed Sid. Luckily they like the idea. Jack throws himself in, deciding to play all the good guys while Billy is the stooge. Billy doesn't realise he's the dragon, but he's giving a fair crack at thwarting the broomstick as Jack tries valiantly to swoop back and forth across the room with theatrical 'Is there rOOOOm on the brOOOOm for a beast like me's.

I could point out that there isn't much room at all for anyone else, but everyone can plainly see that already. The room is pretty crammed with us all in it, plus the plastic 'peep peep' till and assorted 'shop' items. If anyone should urgently need a copy of *Fix it Duck*, a crumpled pile of muslins or a Percy Pig rattle, then we're just the place for them! There's everything here, we're a one-stop shop for all your squashed raisin, cuddly toy and cabbage leaf needs. (I read that a frozen Savoy cabbage leaf is just the ticket for sore nipples. When they're *that* sore you'll try anything. Once.)

The big boys seem happily ensconced in their game so now it is Sid's turn for attention, a fact that he is keenly pointing out. If anyone's going to hear the grand finale about the shower-equipped broomstick, I'd better feed him on the double. I scoop him up, his cheek turns expertly into my chest and his mouth does that expectant goldfish thing, making round lipped 'O' 'O' 'O's as if to say 'At last. What took you so long? A fella could expire with hunger round here.'

Jack is now being the pig. *Is* there a pig in *Room on the Broom*? I don't think so, but he is being a pig anyhow. He performs a sweeping sofa fly past on his hoover attachment broom, flips purposefully around and clobbers the two-year-old dragon, who immediately starts to cry.

'Jack!' I berate in the most convincing authoritative voice I can muster from sitting position with partially exposed breasts and a piranha at my nipple.

'It wasn't me!' says our witch/pig/cat-amongst-the pigeons before slinking guiltily towards the door and, 'Whoops he was gone.'

But not before the furious dragon's pulled himself to his feet, shrieked the shriek of the unjustly tripped, and whacked him fierily broadside. There's a pig trotter here, a dragon talon there and a cacophony of beastly-sounding squawks. I'm sure Julia Donaldson could think of all sorts of imaginative ways to describe it, but things are starting to look nasty, and I for one am not about to sit back and watch poetry in motion.

I slip a furious little finger between my nipple and Sid's vice-like tongue, stride over and into the affray. One boob is hanging out and the baby is going purple with rage. Billy pursues the pig intending, just this once, to have sausage without chips. Jack reels back on him, with a sidelong look at me as though to warn 'Buzz off, that's *my* dragon!' I wade into it regardless, with a face uglier than any Scheffler-drawn baddie and before I can say 'Iggety, ziggety, zaggety zoom', the doorbell rings with such magnificently bad timing I could weep.

I sweep the suddenly cowed children with a glacial look, tuck my boob back into the unhooked cup of my bra and flounce off to answer the door. I open it. I realise milk is leaking from the abandoned nipple in a deep crimson flower across my faded claret top. My face goes scarlet in sympathy. I'm unsure if it's embarrassment or anger, but one way or another I think I'm seeing red.

Five Steps of Anger Management; Taming the Lion Within

If you ever find yourself incandescent with rage at your children, your absent other half, or your treacherously leaky mammary glands, you may want to learn these steps and integrate them into your life.

1) Admit that you are angry, to yourself and/or to someone else.

Practise this response:

'See this red face, right? And this wet top, right? That's anger that is. Grrr!'

Of course, this only works if the person you're angry with is in the same room. Unless you wish to Skype your anger across the continents.

2) Believe you can control your anger. Tell yourself that you can!

   'I will not cry, I will not cry, I will not cry.'

3) Calm down. Control your emotions. Take some time for yourself, breathe deeply, count to ten, cry ... do whatever works for you.

   'Oh, perhaps I *will* cry then.'

4) Decide how to solve the problem. This step only works once you are calm. Figure out what you need and what is fair.

   'Erm. Can I phone a friend?'

5) Express yourself assertively. Ask for what you need. Speak calmly, without yelling, and people will listen to you.

   'Children, you *need* to stop swiping at each other.'

   'Children, *I said* you need to stop swiping at each other.'

   'Please?'

   'Dirk, you *need* to ... oh, you're not there. Shall I write?'

I wonder if I could send a poison pen letter to deepest Africa just to get my own back. Or a poison email? Let's make it a bit more twenty-first century, after all, he is in Telecoms. Or, I dunno, do they still have dragons in deepest Africa? Maybe I should just go the whole hog and contract a fire-breathing baddie to track him down and have Businessman With or Without Chips. He'll be the one on the BA broom, *definitely* without the cat, the dog, the bird, the frog, or three small boys because they're all here at home with me. A long way away. Without him.

Sorry, am I coming across as grumpy? Well, as it happens I am. I am home, effectively alone with a menagerie of juvenile offenders. The house and our lives are chaos. I'm shattered and the boiler's broken down. I, somewhere and at some point, agreed on the dotted line to be the one at home. So therefore sorting out bust boilers is my department on top of everything else. As long as I don't personally boil over with rage before the day is through everything should be fine.

We've been married over ten years now and everything is perfectly happy. Really. (Poison pen letters apart.) It's just that sometimes it can be a bit stressful. We had all those fancy-free years together without kids. We worked, we played, we were on a level footing. Everything was just dandy and oh, if I had only appreciated it. Because once we had kids, suddenly everything changed. And today is one of those days when I wonder if it was for the better.

'Er, hello. Mrs Mo ...'

'Yeah, hello. Come in. Sorry, it's a bit, er chaotic.'

'Oh, not to worry, I've seen all sorts.'

I bet you have. Although I'm pleased to note you're keeping your eyes well above my sopping breast area.

'Whaaaa.'

'Hungry?'

'Too right. Didn't get time for my breakfast yet. The boiler's this way.'

'Cup of tea?'

'Lovely.'

We are on holiday in a cottage in rural Dorset. The main players are huddled around a low coffee table. The heating is on. Rain is lashing at the windows. Jack holds a fistful of cards, instinctively to his chest. Billy has *his* cards laid out plain as day on the surface in front of him. Sid is exploring the skirting boards. Perhaps he is looking for the switch to turn on 'Summer'. I couldn't find anything in the Visitors' Manual when I looked, mind.

I have Mr Stitch the Tailor and Miss Stitch the Tailor's

daughter. I have Master Chop the Butcher's son, Mrs Pill the Chemist's wife and Miss Sole the Fishmonger's daughter. I know that Billy has Mrs Stitch the Tailor's wife. I know that because I can see her on the table in front of me. But I have to pretend I haven't seen her and I ask if he has Master Stitch instead. Which he doesn't. Which I already knew. It is a complex game.

Rules of Happy Families

- Sometimes this game is known as Go Fish. Or at other times Go Wish You Could Shuffle the Cards and Start Again.
- Number of players: 3 or more. Sometimes 5.
- Object of Game: to gather together one coherent and happy family.

1) Shuffle and deal all of the cards face down.
2) The players look at their hands and decide which sort of family they would like. NB: some of the cards in this pack have been updated to suit the times.
   For example there is:
   - Mr Football, the Premiership A-lister whose counterpart is Mrs Football, the WAG and wannabe pop star (ability to sing not necessary).
   - Mr Brushski, the Polish painter-cum-window cleaner whose counterpart is Mrs Brushski the cleaner. Could turn her hand to chimney sweeping if required and will, you can be sure, work jolly hardski at it.
   - Mr Burberry, the Chav whose counterpart isn't his Mrs And whose Burberry is not Burberry either.
   - Mr Telephone, the Telecoms Man whose counterpart is Mrs Permanently-at-the-Other-End-of-the-Telephone, the Telecoms Wife. They have a team of little pint-sized Telecoms. The

omission of a little Miss and the addition of a couple of extra Masters shows the hole in the plan for those who are paying attention, but this is a mere detail.

3) The player to the left of the dealer might start by asking:

'Can I do a swap with Mrs Bun the Baker? *His* hours are tough, but at least he's home for bath time.'

The next player along might then say:

'If you hop off with Mr Bun, then I might leave with Mrs Bung the Brewer. I'd never be back for bath time or indeed before last orders and then where would you be?'

The first player might say:

'Boo', 'hiss' and 'you can iron your own shirts then'.

The second player might respond by saying:

'What, you mean like I always do anyway, then?'

The first player might launch back into another round of:

'Boo' and 'hiss'.

And then the next player along might say:

'Mummy? Daddy? I'm a bit confused. Can we just play the game the way it's *supposed* to go?'

4) The players then resume the game with Mr Telephone the Telecoms Man clocking up some more Air Miles, working his butt off to support Mrs Telephone the Telecoms Wife who stays safely at home cooking, cleaning and looking after their brood of tiny Telecoms.

5) The player whose turn it is next asks another player for a specific card. Mrs Telephone the Telecoms Wife wants the 'Mrs Valued the Individual' card *as well* as the 'Mrs Domestic Goddess the Perfect Mum' card. She wants a lot, it is fair to say.

6) If the player asked has the card it must be handed over and the asker continues to ask for more, even though she seemingly has quite a lot already. Mrs Telephone the Telecoms Wife wanted to be 'at home' with her little ones.

And she got what she wanted. But now she is also sometimes cross at finding herself in this position. She looks at Mr Mackintosh the Briefcase Man, at Miss To-Die-For Heels the City Exec and at Mrs Mobile, the Woman with Purpose all hurrying past her window and she sighs.

7) If the asked player does not understand what his wife really wants and sometimes feels confused, one can perhaps begin to sympathise when he responds by saying 'not at home' and letting the turn pass on.

At the end of the game, the winner is ... well, there is no winner. But players that manage to work through all this, accept and/or modify their lot and jolly well get on with it are on their way to a completed happy family.

Dirk comes back from an all-weeker to Namibia after I've put the boys to bed. He trips over a scooter, which has been left lying broadside in the hallway. There is washing hanging from the banisters. A heap of catalogues and mail teeters on the kitchen worktop like a multicoloured paper tower of Pisa.

'So, how was it?' I ask, 'Namibia?'

'OK,' he mumbles, but he doesn't want to talk about work. He wants to switch off. 'How've they been?'

And I think, not the best actually. We seem to have been enacting the juicier scenes from *Fight Club* most of the week. Everyone has been sick. And we've all been sleeping appallingly. I've had a run of those nights sharing the bed with a hot and restless body jostling in behind me. Not my absent other half getting frisky. A son usually. No, two. Bad dreams. Coughs. Calpol. Sid awake, still needing lots of night-time feeds. And then up at dawn under the impression that 5 a.m. is the new 7 a.m. Every morning. It shouldn't be allowed.

'Oh, fine.' I lie.

He picks up the pile of post. The catalogue on the bottom has stuck to the worktop where some spilt milk must have glued it down a couple of days ago. He frowns and looks at me again 'Look, are you sure you're OK? Do you want extra help? An au pair?' This does not bode well. It means he has seen through my 'fine'. It means he thinks I am not coping.

But I really do not. Want other people in. It would feel like an admission of failure. I gave up my career to do this. I want to do it right. Only it doesn't seem to come out one hundred per cent right all of the time. We get by and some days we have fun. But other days I'm finding it hard to keep on top of everything. And the last thing I want is an extra witness to my chaos. A witness to my shame. Shame at wanting to bite the hand that feeds me, shame at feeling like I am failing and shame at not seeming more grateful than I should at this very moment.

Sometimes I wonder how things would've turned out. If I'd gone back to work. The kids in full-time nursery: 'eight till late'. Or taking in that au pair? But I know in my heart of hearts that it wouldn't be right. To relinquish my kids to the care of someone so young. For so long and so soon. What with their dad being away half the time too. It might suit others, but it wouldn't be my cup of tea.

'No, really, it's fine. Just been a bit tough this week, but I'll be fine.'

And I resolve that I will. Manage just fine. I made the decision to stay at home and devote myself to my family. Therefore I will pull through the new-baby-and-double-toddler fug, take a deep breath and get on with it, try to relax and just enjoy. And I will start by sorting out the mail mountain. Which is essentially what I spend my days doing, anyway, but not with a pile of post.

• • •

It is spring. This time he is in Tanzania. I've had one of those 'must get out of the house before I kill someone' moments. If Dirk *had* returned from Tanzania, laden with homecoming gifts and found one of the recipients dead, I don't think it would have gone down too well. 'Sorry, darling. I was just having one of those days. It started at dawn with Billy falling out of bed and just carried on from there, really. You know, the usual: bickering over who gets the Pingu bowl, squabbles over who sits next to Mummy (no one wanted to), spoon too shiny, milk too milky, bowl upturned and Shreddies dripping onto the floor. It was either crying over the spilt milk or taking the empty bowl and ramming it over his head. Maybe a bit too forcefully.'

Luckily, on this occasion, I had bitten back the urge to lamp him with the Pingu Bowl. (I used to be such a passive sort of person, I'm sure.) I had taken a deep breath, put the bowl down and mopped up the cereal mush with only minimal grumbling. Then I had gathered everyone together, strapped us into duck formation and prepared to go out.

I had solved the unsolvable transportation issue with the help of a buggy board and a borrowed BabyBjörn sling. Passersby look on with a mixture of pity and abject horror at this skewed apparition of a mother and her troop of ducklings. We are a dead ringer for one of those classic pull-along toys of old, except that we've got it slightly wrong. Instead of me being in the lead, we've inverted ourselves. I am at the back of the ascending height-order line and *they* appear to be dragging *me*. Billy is at the front, sitting in the buggy, coming over as the smallest of all. Jack is next, standing, face forward atop the buggy board. Then comes Sid, facing me, snuggled up in the sling. Last but not least there's me, bringing up the rear, the tallest and probably tiredest of all as I push and carry the whole little merry-go-round forth. I am sure half of Highbury must think I'm quackers. Still, it works for me and it gets me out of the house.

I hustle everyone on towards the playground. Kids are running. Mothers are drinking coffee from cardboard cups in corrugated shrugs. A couple of teenagers slouch in the shelter and the swings groan pitifully, crying out for oil. I know how they feel.

Sid is dozing in the sling while I push the other two round on the bicycle roundabout. I never liked roundabouts at the best of times, but trying to hoik my own not inconsiderable adult weight around it with a growing baby strapped to my front was never going to be in any way easy.

I stop for a breather. The lads skitter off to the slide. I sit down, puffing, and enjoy the moment of peace before Sid wakes up and requires a feed. At least in here I can do it without fear of an old bloke telling me to go and breastfeed somewhere else. Like in the playground loo. Which as it happens ought to have a health warning slapped onto its door. Tempting prospect.

Sid wakes. I feed him. At the edge of the sandpit, not in the loo. Contented, he looks back up at me, the soft downy hair on his apple cheek catching the light and causing my breath to snag. I smile, gulping in the gossamer beautiful, mother-rush love. And then we get up, I round up the others and we are off again on our travels.

Scene opens in a courtroom with a judge, a clerk of the court and a defence counsel in a semicircle facing the audience. The jury sits to one side and the defendant is in the witness box.

JUDGE: Ladies and gentlemen of the Jury, have you reached a verdict?

JURY
FOREMAN: We have m'lud.

JUDGE: And how do you find the defendant?

FOREMAN: Guilty on every count!

(An audible gasp is heard from the Visitors' Gallery. The defendant lowers her head.)

JUDGE: Then there is nothing to do but pass sentence. Ladies and gentleman, on this day Charlotte Moerman, a 'Full-Time Mother', has been found guilty in court under the Feeling Guilty Act.

Guilt at leaving behind everything offered on a plate in terms of education and opportunities.

Guilt at choosing in their stead a life of chickenpox, nits and avocado mush.

Guilt at leaving behind a career.

Guilt at *wanting* to leave behind a career.

Guilt at realising that on regular occasions, she is actually not very good at her chosen path, this full-time mothering thing.

Guilt at feeling cross or sad or both at herself, and her largely innocent other half when in fact this is what *she* wanted and she should be jolly well grateful.

The accused is to be taken from this place and made to feel permanently guilty for now and ever more.

(More gasps from the Visitors' Gallery. The defendant looks up, eyes glistening.)

COUNSEL: Objection m' Lud.

JUDGE: Objection overruled. Mrs Moerman. Do you have anything to add?

DEFENDANT: Yes m'lud. Guilty as charged.

Chapter 13

Later. Much, much later, we are all gathered on the sofa watching *Sam and Mark's Guide to Dodging Disaster*. The presenters are runners up from *Pop Idol* 2003. When they bowed out to the eventual winner I was pregnant with Billy, and Sid was but a twinkle in his daddy's eye. At the time they were probably gutted. But now that their victor has faded into oblivion (Michelle McWho?) and they've shown they have the CBBC Factor, they must feel as though the world is their oyster. Albeit it a rather hair-raising one at times.

'Look!' giggles Jack as a lion marks his territory on the blond one who is trying to hide in the bushes. ('Mark by name, Marked by nature,' says the Voiceover Man though I think I'd be narked by nature myself, wouldn't you?)

'Oh no!' squeals Billy, thrilled but petrified enough to flee to the safety of the stairs as they are later charged by a big burly bad-tempered bison.

The programme is a guide to surviving the most dangerous situations that Mother Nature can chuck at you. Because, let's face it, it is useful to know how to deal with an attacking baboon on the wild old streets of Highbury. Especially, but not exclusively, on a match day.

I snuggle closer into Sid, and Dirk extends his arm across the back of the sofa around us both. We watch as the next big disaster unfolds. We can't wait for their hammed-up responses – plenty of screaming, face-pulling and the occasional smelly sock. Today they are in North Africa, where they find themselves in a sandstorm. I can almost imagine myself there in their place.

The scene would be of a mummy driving in her car, all set for a lovely picnic lunch in the sun. The sky is blue. The sands are white. She has the radio on and is singing along, bopping her head to the beat. Not a care in the world. Totally unsuspecting. The Voiceover Man suggests she might like to tune in to a different channel to check for storm warnings. But no, she'd prefer to just chunter along regardless, enjoying her own choice of tune instead.

Then the wind picks up and sand starts to fly. Small granules at first. And then the storm really hits. It is not what she expected from her jolly drive out at all. This is no picnic. She's getting buffeted about from all sides, and the grains are starting to feel abrasive. She's getting a bit hacked off and there is sand in her sandwich too! Peeved would be a good way to describe her right now. She screams and pulls a face. There is a very real danger that the wind could turn and she might get stuck with the face of a griper. There is also a danger that people might get hurt or even drawn apart whilst the visibility remains so poor.

Luckily, Voiceover Man is there to help. If you get caught in a storm like this, remember these rules:

1) Find yourself some shelter. And don't let yourself get buried. The storm will abate in time and you'll find yourself much better able to get back on top of things if you haven't let yourself get bogged down with junior bed-bouncing competitions that always end in tears, Tyson-style fights being played out in the living room (Myson versus Myson),

and werewolf-like baying at your other half when the moon comes out. Or the sun, alternatively.

2) Lie on the ground, and keep your eyes, ears and nose covered at all times. In other words, don't let it get up your nose. Put your arms over your head to protect it from objects being hurled by the strength of the storm. Those Julia Donaldson board books do seem to have a habit of getting themselves airborne.

3) Wear appropriate protection. Make a conscious effort to put on a silly animal mask or have 'princess eyelashes' painted around your eyes. Sometimes on your chin. They won't make the nasty bits vanish, but being Princess for a while can never fail to improve your day.

4) Do not split up. In the thick of it all, you can easily lose your partner. Don't get separated, and make sure you hold on tight, won't you? Because, in the words of a Voiceover Woman I once knew, he's worth it.

5) Keep an eye on the horizon. Concentrate on getting through to the other side. It is not going to last for ever so keep your head down until the sandstorm passes over and you should be all right.

It is all sound advice from Voiceover Man. He knows what he is talking about. Because the storm does pass over. Sam and Mark, as they always do, return to being cheeky chappies, relaxing back at home with broad smiles and a mug of tea in each hand. And our mummy too, she pulls through the worst and her smile finds its way back onto her face. For most of the time at least.

There are days that I feel quite lost in spite of travelling round endlessly familiar local circles and routines. And there are days when I feel consumed with guilt at the ugly feelings that occasionally surface in spite of living a life of luck on a plate. I wonder sometimes that I am not visited by plagues or spectres in the night. I do not deserve my good fortune.

But then the dark, helpless moments become fewer and further between. A chuckle erupts that warms me to the core. A small hot hand creeps into mine and stays there. A generous kiss bursts on my denim-clad bottom. An anti-dandruff shampoo ad is spontaneously finished off with a genius echo of 'knees and toes, knees and toes'.

These are the times when I feel happy and proud of my gaggle of lads. Appreciative and tender, like I should be all the time. I am lucky to have them with me. Jack and Sid, an arm's reach away, there when I want or need to hold them. And Billy, now fully recovered with a clean bill of health. So different to how things might've been.

They are there for me to bear-hug at will. To teach and shape and have fun with. To be pirates with. To be a Thunderbird with. And to engage with in the game where they repeat everything I say where they repeat everything I say, except 'I am a girl and I love Barbies!' or 'mushrooms are yummy!' just say. And I am also lucky, I think, to be able to play imaginary I-Spy games with them too.

'I spy with my little eye something beginning with ... S!'

'Sid?'

'No.'

Sunshine?'

'No.'

'Satsuma?'

'No. You'll never get it!'

'Oh go on then, I give up. What is it?'

'Sircus!'

'But you actually have to see it. That's the whole point. There isn't a circus in this room is there?'

'So! It's what I was thinking about!'

'And circus doesn't begin with S either.'

'Doesn't matter. It's what I was thinking that counts.'

The truth is I revel in the kudos of having three pre-school kids and everything that they bring.

'You're the best mummy in the world' they have been known to say on occasion, i.e., more than once. I only wish I really was.

It is summer 2006. Jack is now nearly four, Billy is going on two and half, and Sid is about six months. I have emerged from the fug. Time has moved on, I have made my way through, and it did not cross my mind at all to try to find the receipt and see if I could take them back to the shop. (Well, maybe not more than once or twice.) I did not turn into a permanently irritable old cow either. And I did not resort to throwing my hands in the air with an exaggerated Gallic shrug and say 'Oh fug it.' But phew, there were some moments, all the same.

Thank goodness that is all behind me now. No? I will never again wake up and think, horror, my house has transformed into Bedlam. It will never cross my mind to wonder if my husband has left us for a safely distant camel. I will never think, blimey it is all too much and take on the advice of that Boogie Beebies guy and curl myself up in a ball, make myself small and take solace in the fact that he, at least, thinks I did great today. Nope, none of that because Things are Getting Better and I live in hope that the worst of the chaos is over. ('Ha ha, famous last words,' says the nearby mother of teenagers ...)

Everything feels different now. Jack is fast approaching school. Billy is fast approaching pre-school. And Sid is fast approaching being pigeon-holed as the cheeky chappy joker. I'm not sure if it's his two-tone eye, half brown, half blue, that makes you look again, his strange resemblance to Graham Norton, or just the fact that as the baby of the family we all laugh indulgently at him whether he's just spilled custard all down his front, chuckled like his carry-on namesake, or mischievously flicked Petits Filous at the face of one of his brothers. 'Aaah, would you look at Sid, bless him?'

Of course, I still do all the stuff that you have to do. I wash, I tidy and I churn out food that I hope might float their boat. Still no scrambled eggs or mushrooms of course. But 'bacon cake' (quiche), green beans (!), Branston pickle sandwiches and boiled egg with soldiers made from bagels. Not sure what the Grand Old Duke of York would make of a regiment of round-shouldered (bent?) troops but my boys think they're the bees' knees.

Dirk meanwhile comes and goes and we all try to catch a slice of him before he's gone again. For the boys, there's no looking back the moment his key is in the door. They are in seventh heaven when he steps in, plonks his codjecar on the floor and waits, arms outstretched for the onslaught to arrive. They wash up at his feet and buffet him for hugs, airport presents and permission to skip their bath. I wait in turn for my hug, a fresh pile of well-travelled laundry and permission to skip bedtime stories.

I am delighted to see my husband, of course. In spite of the occasional little grumble, which I'm sure you wouldn't begrudge me, I would like to resolutely point out that I love him very much. I crave his company. I crave his in-the-flesh, grown-up, end-of-the-day conversation. And his authoritative refereeing skills tend to come in handy on occasions too. I, in turn, think (hope?) he still enjoys my company. I hold fast in my conviction that he does not consider me the stroppy baggage wifey back at home. Really.

But even so, as they always do, cravings come with a double-edged sword. Mine is to feel a little cast out in the cold while our returning hero nods appreciatively, and accepts the mantle of adoring sons who bring slippers to his feet and ringed Lego Club catalogues to his fingers. They do not quite go as far as to bring out a portly toy-farm Friesian calf, but they might as well do.

Still, thinking what Voiceover Man might advise, I know I must not try to compete. We are not in the *Big Brother* house, bitching, blinkered and hell-bent on being the longest to avoid going out to chat with Davina. We are not competing for the love of our children (even though sometimes. Just sometimes. It seems like they love him more than me). We are trying to be the best parental double-act that we can possibly be.

'Those who play team sports usually have a ball,' Voiceover Man might sagaciously say. How wise. Perhaps I just need to remember that one. We are both on the same side.

We have some time out. Together. Sans enfants. We stay in an old coaching inn with only a handful of rooms. We sleep in a bed that does not have Calpol, Lego and discarded stickers littering the bedhead.

We go for a walk by a river, striding through knee-deep grass whilst nearby sheep pause to watch and consider our progress. At a nettle-dense bridge, he reaches for my hand to help me negotiate the overgrown bottom step. We meander past a pebbly beach, carved out by the curve of the river, and we say how the boys would love it here.

I squeeze Dirk's hand and we walk on, tramping along companionably. We reach a field with a 'Warning Bull' sign. We make a dash for it to the other side, giggling. We make it, out of breath, but uninjured. We leave the fields and the bad-tempered bulls behind us, no longer quite so empty.

My husband asks for an axe for Christmas. It is an unusual choice. I wonder if the grinding of my teeth could be heard above the roar of the aeroplane engines all the way up at 35,000 feet. Gulp. I really did not mean it.

With my marriage I got a new name and a dress. I also got a husband I am really rather fond of. OK, so I grumbled a bit … sometimes more than a bit … when I was home alone with the Smalls. And perhaps even now there is the odd frown when they spat, or bung a whole toilet roll down the loo, or 'lose' their shoes, or exude blood-curdling torture-chamber shrieks (at the table sometimes too), or make me shout even though I DON'T LIKE SHOUTING.

But I wouldn't change anything for the world. I am quite aware that we went into this together. He is doing his best for us, yet, ingrate that I am, I occasionally choose him as the scapegoat for my frustrations. I will just have to show him my love with my actions. Respond to his call and axe him to forgive me.

So I buy him the axe. I am sold, in fact, a whopping great lumberjack's hatchet by the guy in the hardware shop who must be wetting himself in the stock room, egged on by his mates to try selling the most ridiculous item of the day to the gullible broad out front.

'It is for chopping wood,' he assures me. And I take it and stash it under the buggy and I even go into Halifax to pay in a cheque straight afterwards. I am lucky that I am not arrested. It certainly makes for an arresting beribboned package under the tree. Dirk opens it gamely, explains later on that it is probably for chopping wood in a forest, with very big old gnarly trees in it. Not for the rather tamer firewood-splitting job that he had had in mind for keeping our home fires burning.

He takes the axe back and swaps it for a smaller one. I am quite relieved actually. But perhaps that is all he had wanted. I have learned my lesson.

I go out for a drink with the NCT gang. They are all in stitches over the axe story. I, fortunately, am not. In stitches, that is.

Every two or three months we have a girls' night out. A bite to eat here, a glass of wine there, and the chance to do as the wonderful Frankie once suggested and just relax. I'm one of a weekly Starbucks coffee posse. And two or three times a year, I also catch up with Claudia, Pippa and Charlotte. Between us we now have a total of seven children. We no longer dance to the strains of Salt 'n Pepa, and we have clearly been ignoring their suggestion to merely talk about sex. Even the one amongst us without a child must've been guilty of it at least once or twice I'd wager.

Occasionally, just occasionally, I also meet up with old friends and colleagues from the time Before Children – Friends Reunited, former colleagues' leaving dos, ex-BA meet-ups to compare notes on what everyone went on to do next. I try not to guffaw and/or stamp on my interlocutor's toes when they ask 'So, Charlotte. Tell me, are you *working* these days?'

Many of these friends from Times Past have yet to the make the big jump themselves. It is good to see them. Good to catch up. But even so, I wonder if I am too different for them now. Amongst the childless I often detect what I think of as the Platform 9¾ effect. You've either pushed your luggage trolley through the brick wall portal or you haven't. (Perhaps this is what Dad was referring to?) Those who haven't just don't get the magic and the madness on the other side of the divide.

We live alongside the Muggles, but they fail to see or understand us.

If pressed on the matter, they look at us with undisguised horror as though to say: 'If *I* look at platform 9 or thereabouts, all I see is a drunk guy eating a burger, and a exasperated businessman, cussing because he's missed the 21.47 to Letchworth. No I'm sorry, I just don't see the magic.'

Luckily, there are plenty around who *do* see it and are indeed keen to share and commiserate. I am now a fledgling member of the Highbury Mums' Mafia. We drink prodigious quantities of coffee by day. We drink prodigious quantities of wine by night. We hold our Cosa Nostra mob meetings in Il Bacio's Pizzeria or up the road at the Highbury Barn pub. Or failing that, we meet in someone's house for what is loosely termed our 'book group' where we sometimes manage to spend at least ten minutes discussing the text.

And then that is it. We boomerang back onto how everyone is or is not coping with the task of dragging up our children. We are unable to help ourselves. We go over our failures with a mixture of mortification and devil-may-care glee. For some, it is a bearing and sharing process, a kind of 'Mums Anonymous' for the relief of pains (usually those in the bum). For others, they rather pride themselves on the subject; if you excel at something you might as well admit it. It is almost as competitive as who had the worst labour. But not quite.

FIRST MUM: Well, guess what? They've only broken another window!
ANOTHER: Another?
FIRST MUM: Yup. We've now broken eight windows in total in our house, plus one of the neighbours'. When I enquired as to how the window might

	have been cracked, the boys racked their brains and then said the only *unlikely* possibility was when they were playing cricket in that room.
ANOTHER:	Blimey, well that's not what I'd call cricket!
YET ANOTHER:	(*possibly me*) Well, I nearly lost the plot when mine left the tap running in the sink above our kitchen. The sink without an overflow. The kitchen with the newly replastered ceiling. That isn't very new-looking any more.
ANOTHER:	Ooh, that must've put the dampeners on the kitchen renovations!
FIRST MUM:	(*clearly warming up to it now*) Well, we've had a plaster disaster too – when the halogen lights fused and a dark stain arrived on the dining room ceiling the time everyone was having *so* much fun splashing in the bathroom above. And then there were the fires. We've had two of them in our bedroom, both caused in the same way and five years apart – a rogue pillow fighter leaving his pillow over a lamp that had been knocked onto the bed in the fray. It wasn't a pretty sight. And the smell wasn't too great either.'
ANOTHER:	Hmm. Bet there wasn't much in the way of sweet pillow talk in your house *that* night. Or the time after.
YET ANOTHER:	Well, we had our front bay window smashed from the inside. They were surfing on a back-to-front armchair. Most probably drunk at the time. Headbanging to Black Sabbath. The naughty step was on full active service for quite some time after that one I can promise you.'

ANOTHER: Terrible. Taste in music I mean.
FIRST MUM: When mine peed in the waste paper basket, I
             nearly peed on him.

House point to the family Lloyd duly allocated there I think.

Jack comes to me and says 'Mummy, I'm going to marry you when you're dead because I love you'. The sentiment is all good, so it just wouldn't be right to quibble on the detail.

I cuddle him close into me and kiss him on his brow. Billy, sensing a love-in in the offing, bundles himself over, removes both my slippers and starts exaggeratedly tickling my stockinged feet. 'Tiggle tiggle tiggle.' (It is a tricky one to say when you are small and very excited.)

'Ooh. Ooh. Stop it!' I say, because that is what I am required to do. But I don't want him to stop because it is delicious. Jack's now joining in the tussle, fingers hovering and ready for action. They are chuckling insanely. Is there a Nobel Prize for Chuckling? If not, perhaps there should be. Otherwise I would give them the Nobel Prize for Peace. Not as in quiet.

More as in restoring it. To me.

Sid, not to be outdone, is sitting in the baby bouncer gurgling with sheer delight. He is flapping his arms like a birdman in a human flying competition, launching himself optimistically off a Victorian pier. I notice that he has managed to squirrel into his hand the leaflet from the top of the pile of post that I had brought in here to process before it glued itself to the kitchen worktop. I remove the avid ticklers from about my person, and reach to grab it from his hand before he starts to chew it.

It is a flier for roving computer repairs. 'Fast reliable service!' it says. 'Free estimate!' 'Hardware replacements and recovery of lost data or files!'

I pop a rattle into Sid's now empty hand and reflect that today, at least, is a good day. I set aside the flier for recycling and smile as I recline back into the Tickle Club. This is what is making me happy. Tickles. Laughter ringing out *loud*. And the realisation that I have recovered some very important lost data.

I consider ringing the number on the flier to tell them that offering restoration services to the mother board might also be lucrative. But then again, on balance, I think better of it.

Sometimes I feel a bit like the small brown and ordinary mouse in *The Gruffalo*. I am quietly trying to find my way, minding my own business really, but I've got this deep dark and scary wood to negotiate. There are all sorts of treats to be had if I forage in the right places. But I am also never quite sure what's going to pop up next. I need to keep my wits about me and do my best to avoid being eaten up by the sheer overwhelming enormity of life at home with three small boys and a frequently absent husband.

I'd thought that the grass was greener before I entered into this wood. I arrived all full of hope. My nose twitched in anticipation. My mouth turned up at the corners in an expectant Scheffler-style grin. But, hang on, what was this? A whole host of baddies lying in wait for me? Oodles of them. Often hunting in packs.

There is Guilt. Ooh, he's a mean-looking fella. Prickly with spikes running all down his back. And nobbly boils too. Then there's Exhaustion. What a rotter he turned out to be. Four arms and six legs, all tickly and green. Bitterness. A proper nasty piece of work. Tentacles, pointed teeth and the evilest frown you've *ever* seen. Loneliness – he's drawn in squiggly black felt tip. Frustration – he's the one who growls. And Stress – he's got a long wriggly tail and eyes on stalks. Lots of them.

Some days they make me feel really bad. Ever so not on top of things. And then other days I rally and Hope, Joy and Play-Doh contrive to get me back on track. For a little while. Until the little beasties come out of their hiding places and join in the affray.

There's my old friend the Fox. That would be Jack. He's cuddly for sure. And clever and handsome too. He's the urban variety who lives happily alongside us all for the most part, but has a few villainous tricks up his sleeve when you turn your back. He is a terror for wiping his snout on his sleeve. He is a dab hand at turning tail and bunny-hopping his scooter, usually right into my shins. And the shoes he does them in are so scuffed, Imelda Marcos would weep. (Or just tell him to put on another pair.)

If Jack asked me to come and have lunch in his underground house, I would have to insist that he wiped his nose (on a tissue) first and promised that the toilet seat within had been left Very Correctly down. I would also be keen to find out if he had hung his coat up properly and hadn't abandoned his shoes on the stairs where I might just happen to trip over them in the dark. As has happened. More than once. (Bare-buttock sliding down the carpeted stairs, sending my slippers into orbit with my nightie round my armpits was not a good look. And it felt pretty painful too.)

Billy would be the Owl. He watches from a safe distance until the time is right, then swoops. He will silently sabotage one of Jack's puzzles or games, and make silent flight before anyone's twigged. He becomes most active at twilight, kicking off his habitual barrage of 'Why's just when he should be settling down for the night. And he helps by stealth, taking items from the supermarket shopping and hiding them in the places you'd least expect – Ribena in the wine rack, milk in the dishwasher, eye make-up remover in the fridge. Sometimes, as I undo all his 'help', I wonder if Billy's posted my head somewhere temporarily irretrievable too.

If Billy asked me to come and have lunch in his treetop house, I would have to insist that he asked me again with a nice please rather than whingeing, thank you very much. I would also be keen to obtain a promise that he would not mess up the sofa just when I was planning to sit down on it for five minutes. And I would need to get a full brief of what he was expecting of me once I got inside so that we'd avoid unpleasant scenes such as me sitting in the wrong place, saying the wrong thing, having the wrong face or whatever. Treetop house mix-ups can frequently happen without proper upfront thinking. Just ask WoL.

That leaves Sid, who would of course be the Snake. He spends much of his time slithering around the floor, acting the wriggly livewire. His saliva-dripping tongue, though admittedly not forked, spends an inordinate amount of time hanging serpent-like from his mouth. And he likes to camouflage himself from loose-cannon older brothers by the cunning strategy of blinking his eyes tightly shut, and the less cunning one of playing peek-a-boo behind the curtain – works fine until a mistimed 'boo' breaks his cover.

If Sid asked me to come and have lunch in his log-pile house, I would have to insist that I already spend far too much time in the company of him and his logs. If pressed, however, I would acquiesce on the proviso that he doesn't have a hissy fit if I get in the way of him propelling himself down the stairs again. (Spoilsport that I am.) Or that he would not try to slough me off when I endeavour to put him in the buggy doing that backward banana thing. Enough to drive anyone wild.

Looked at in their entirety, they are a motley crew. But it is impossible nonetheless not to fall for their charms. And besides, we all know that good old Mouse wins the day and the little beasties toe the line in the end. And they all live happily ever after. Hurrah. End of story. Except of course that's not the story in its entirety is it? It actually happens like this:

Our stalwart friend the Mouse, the one who has done all that hard work telling the story and coming up with the genius ideas to navigate through the hairy bits, well, she might start to feel a little sidelined. Because, though the reader's been with her all the way, guess who swans in at the end? He takes all the glory, has the book named after him and doesn't he just look so darn good too? For most of the gig, he's only been present in everyone's imagination. Then at last he puts in an appearance. And look, everyone's in awe. Everything's got much more exciting all of a sudden. Ooh! La-de-Gruffa-la.

But the Mouse, bless her, is a steady and sensible creature. Although she may wrinkle up her rodent nose for a millisecond or two, she knows that far worse things that can happen to a mouse. (She could be sent back onto a caged, spinning treadmill for starters.) The wood might sometimes feel a cold place. Yes, and sometimes her new friend and ally the Gruffalo might sod right off again. Leave her for a Large Bird instead. On the whole, though, she prefers it when he stays. Stops to have tea in her mousey house. Or wine if she can swing it. (Do Gruffalos drink wine? They do if the Mouse says so.)

She gets what she wants in the end this mouse. The nut. The Gruffalo and a measure of satisfaction: job well done. Perhaps the manner of getting there hadn't been quite what she'd envisaged, but they all got there in the end. And surely, that is the point.

Chapter 14

I am feeling slightly loopy. It is a couple of weeks before Jack starts school. Last week, I said I was feeling laid-back about it. The start of a new adventure. Now I am bricking myself. It seems too soon.

As though to make up for the fact that I am shortly to push my first-born out onto the educational treadmill, I am throwing myself into playing his favourite games. It is much more fun than naming socks for starters.

Today we're making an airport on the living-room floor. There are masking-taped roads bringing our Hot Wheels ferried passengers to their flights. The terminal is made from a shoe box, and toilet-roll walkways take our imaginary passengers out to their planes. A plastic ear-bud box is playing the part of a fuel tanker. And there's a hangar, made from upturned plastic teacups supporting a tea-tray roof. Our motley crew of plastic jets and Lego helicopters busily taxi back and forth, and jet off to amazing destinations.

It is high in our top ten of games. As I kneel on the carpet with a mini jumbo in my fist, I wonder if they realise I used to work with real planes in my time. How Dirk spends large chunks of his life in airports such as these, without the masking tape but equally sticky it seems. How wider family and friends have travelled, and still do. I ponder how ironic it is that I am playing a travelling game while grounded firmly on the living-room floor. It is true, I don't get my passport out so much these days, but who needs real travel anyway?

'Flight Number 3. You are cleared for take-off,' says Jack importantly. 'Chocks away!'

'Chocs!' echoes Billy appreciatively.

The boys grab a plane each and *n'yow* them off into the sky. We are competing on who is flying to the most outlandish destination. I suggest I'm off to Marks and Sparks. Billy's going to Holland, Jack to Mars. Sid's keeping it under his hat. The game is going well and I sit back, allowing my plane to refuel. I consider making a cuppa. But then someone grabs someone else's plane, the tea-tray hangar collapses, and the considered tannoy announcements disintegrate into an all-out yell fest.

I distract them with biscuits. They sit on the carpet, sating themselves with apple juice and Hobnobs. Heathrow has had to deal with fog, ice and suitcase drifts before, but never yet biscuit-crumb hailstorms that I am aware of. The black USAF fighter jet doesn't look so cool with rolled-oat dandruff. And it'd better be prepared for a bumpy landing too. Touchdown on that debris-strewn runway will almost certainly not be a piece of cake.

They dispatch the biscuits fast, and then they're up, ready again for more airport action. I guide them through a tour of matchbox Passport Control and Security. Everyone takes their shoes off and puts them back on again. We take in the Control Tower, a multicoloured Duplo masterpiece, and beg the occupants to please not go on strike again today. And then we stop off in Duty Free to eye up an enormous Toblerone the size of a toothpaste box. That is quite big when the planes are the size of a bar of soap.

257

Then Flight Number 3 is suddenly diverted off course to somewhere Under the Sofa. Someone hijacks a sock. The pilot of USAF Biscuit Crumb is trampled in the fray and the noise level shoots up. I silently thank my lucky stars we've used plastic cutlery for the crash barriers and swoop in to save the day with my heroic rescue helicopter. One of the propellers is missing but it doesn't matter because it's got great chopper sound effects and a flashing red light if you press the button. And often if you don't.

I am now the Sky Sheriff. I have a gun (two pointing fingers) and a loud voice. The hijackers are temporarily gobsmacked. They are simple souls, these hijackers. They are not looking for $200 million and the release of a hundred jailed rebel separatists. Being little boys, what they want is food, a good run out every day, guns and plenty of references to poo. So when mummy forgets all her pre-children resolutions about no weaponry in the house and voluntarily pretends to wield a gun, they are tickled pink. When I tell them it is loaded with poo pellets, they practically wet themselves.

'Get those planes back in the sky, I'm tellin ya! I should warn you here and now that I am armed and dung-erous!'

The game kicks back off with fresh verve. We are having a ball, all of us. I spend a good couple of hours making, laying out, playing and keeping the peace. Forget notches on the career ladder, how's that for an afternoon's achievement? I have had fun. I am content. What you seize is what you get in an afternoon at home with the small people.

When we finally knock off for tea the pilots park up their planes in the hangar. USAF BC drifts off to dream about perfectly executed 4 g negative dives and skilfully dodging the odd crummy asteroid storm. And then this version of Heathrow shuts down for the night.

The kitchen, by contrast, is still abuzz with excitement. 'Tomorrow', clamours Jack who is still completely beside himself, 'let's make the moon with craters and spaceships ... and stars and planets with rings and everything! We can all be the aliens, and *you* can be the Space Ranger. With a Mega Patrol Space Blaster that fires out alien poo!'

We are on the brink of something new. The game we have been playing for about four years now will be broadly familiar to many. When you initially log on, there is a loud soundtrack that some might find annoying at first, but you soon get used to it. You are invited to skip the intro if you wish. But don't. You'll realise in time that's a really fun bit.

In the game, Mummy is a Special Agent. She must find her way to the end, fire-fighting along the way and picking up points in the Build a Happy Home Challenge. She must carry her passengers carefully along with her at all times without running out of fuel. She should pick up bonus energy credits where she can along the way, and try not to hit anything. Apart from the baddies that is.

These baddies will try to hamper her progress. If she wants (which she probably doesn't) she can use her imaginary poo gun to pick them off. Otherwise she should hunt out other weapons for brassed-off destruction. Because for the good of mankind, or at least for everyone in her household, she needs to blast away those ugly feelings of inadequacy, guilt and other nasty stuff.

The Special Agent needs to control herself by using the arrow keys. Forward is a good one. Even though sometimes, would you believe it, she might now want to go back! She can use the side arrows to shift lanes. Looking back, she's slalomed all over. Reluctant to leave the Work Lane at first, she soon changed her tune after skidding into the Stay at Home With Kids Lane. Accelerating more than anyone thought possible, she went from zero to three in sixty seconds. When she got there she sometimes looked around in a panic, wondering if there was a Time Out button. Other times she coasted and found it was, wheeee, really good fun!

And now the time has come to think about turning a new direction. The chequered flag on this leg is already beckoning. It is the beginning of the end of something big. The start of something new and daunting, that she's not sure she's ready yet to face. If quizzed, the Special Agent would really rather apply the brakes and stay in the lane she's in. But she can't control the speed of this game. Acceleration is automatic.

Summer swings into autumn. The air is slightly damp. I am walking down the street with Jack's hand in mine. He is wearing hemmed up M&S trousers, a crisp yellow polo shirt and a bottle-green fleece. My last school uniform was bottle-green. I've never been able to wear it since. The colour, not the uniform, though to be fair I haven't tried recently.

After a long summer's wait, it is finally here. The Start of School. I'd say he is fairly ready, aside from a few glitches like learning the name of his new gaff (Jack's convinced he is going to the 'John Lewis' school. There *is* a John in it and we're not talking about the toilet.) But me? I'm a different matter entirely.

I am stressed. The first of my babies is spreading his wings, teetering on the edge, poised and ready to spend the lion's share of his waking hours elsewhere. Last week I said I was fine. Today I am all of a flutter. The trouble is just he's so keen to go.

We've been leading up to this fabled day for weeks. I've named all his kit, I've charged the camera, I've cut his hair and it is fairly straight. We've been poring over the Starting School book all summer. I think he was slightly confused when we first got it. The front cover depicts the title written in giant-size letters. There is a kid dangling from the G, someone clambering through one of the Os, and a little girl hanging onto S for dear life. For a while I'm sure he thought that school was all about alphabet mountaineering.

I am hoping that all our reading of the first-term experiences of Gavin and Errol and Sophie and Sushma and David and Kate and Robert and Alison several times a day will help to assuage first-day nerves. It certainly seems to be working. I am lulling myself into a state of calm by robotically enumerating their names over and over in my head as though counting sheep. And then it occurs to me to wonder how Jack's managing too.

'Everything OK there, love?'

'Fine!' he replies, a right eager beaver.

'Good. Good. And, is there anything you want to go over before we go in? Anything you might be the teensiest bit still worried about?'

He pauses for a while and looks up perplexed 'Well, there is one thing. How will I ever know everyone's names?'

Good point. Gavin and his many mates could seem a daunting example. 'Don't worry. Everyone will take a while,' I explain, 'and you know your own name. That's a good start!'

This seems to satisfy him for now. Then, being a boy, his thoughts skitter off to his privates. 'And what if I can't find the toilets?'

I can see too how this could be worrisome. Toilets are dangerous places. The boys have seen the power that public loos have to transform me from nice Mummy into evil-faced, shouty witch. When one of them heads like a heat-seeking missile to the horror-movie toilet brush, say. Or zooms, as if by magnet, straight to the compelling little open, shut, open, shut door on the top of the sanitary bin. Or, worst of all, reaching up and unlocking the door just when it is finally Mummy's turn on the throne. (Thanks boys.)

'Oh, I wouldn't bog yourself down worrying about that,' I suggest cheerfully. And when he doesn't get it I try 'Just sniff a bit and follow your nose.' He looks at me as though I've gone insane. 'Or otherwise you could just ask the teacher. She's the one whose name you should learn first, by the way.'

Then we turn the corner, and suddenly we've arrived. We're at the school gates. Jack skips in like Julie Andrews on an Austrian film set. I follow rather more reluctantly, like an orphan who is kicking back at the prospect of being decked out in head-to-foot curtains, before the bit where we break into song and decide everything's terribly chipper. We hang around shiftily, uncertain of our territory. Dirk's followed us in with the buggy and the other boys, here as pit-crew support.

The bell rings. The Reception class queues up next to the wall mural of London created by the pupils to celebrate the Millennium. There's the already-old football stadium. There's a number 19 bus. There's Big Ben. Jack edges up close to the famous clock tower, which is comfortingly about 2.5 cm high. Next to some of the decidedly big Reception kids, Jack looks not a lot taller himself.

The teacher comes out to collect us. A huddle of parents trail in with their young. Jack and I follow like urban sheep. I remove Jack's coat and hang it on his pictured peg and we go into the classroom after the self-assured Scarlett who's already been here all of three days. She beelines towards one of half a dozen tables, grabs her name from a pile and pops it into an animal-themed pot in the centre. Kind of like clocking in at the zoo.

'Let's find out which table your name's on shall we?' I suggest encouragingly. 'Oh, here we are. The Giraffe table.' Jack, who from my brief scan in the playground, is one of, if not *the* shortest in the school. Someone who was allocating groups must've surely been having a laugh.

Jack scoops his name, slots it in and makes his way over to the Mobilo corner. Scarlett's already there gathering a pile of red cubes and a stray head. Jack hunkers down next to her with a Duplo camel in hand. I'm not sure what to do. I could hang around, muscle in and tell them my best camel joke. (What do you call a camel with no humps? Humphrey.) Or I could inch off. Leave them to it.

Another little boy I don't recognise joins in. He picks up an axle and a couple of wheels and begins intently building. The teacher makes her way over and kneels down with them, smiling warmly and asking their names. Jack looks up and begins to talk ten to the dozen about his name, his brothers, his shiny new school shoes and the naming of a rabbit called Ronald. The other boy says he has a guinea pig called Frank.

I stand awkwardly, looking on from a height. I am pleased it is going so smoothly. There have been no tears. No histrionics. Not from Jack, either. I am really proud of him. But I also feel a bit deserted. (As in abandoned. Not transformed into something that is needed and wanted by the camel.)

We are allowed to stay with them a little while if we want to. But he seems so sure and capable piecing together plastic bricks with his friends, new and old, that he doesn't really need me. It is gutting but I think it's best if I leave him to it.

I bend down and kiss the crown of his head. 'Bye bye then, big boy.' His eyes barely flicker back to me as he horses around with the camel and his new guinea-pig friend. I see that they are laughing together. I see that he will be OK.

This morning, I felt like I was in a game of Jenga. Someone was about to take a vital piece out and everyone would hold their breath to see if the whole stack would topple over. I withdraw from the classroom and rejoin Dirk and the others. And I realise with a sigh of relief that everything, so far at least, has not come crashing down around us.

Starting School

On the first day, Jack is shown the toilet block. There are *four* small toilets in a row. He realises it would be hard to miss them. Especially as they smell so pongy. (Mummy was right.)

In the Classroom there is a Home Corner, a Book Corner and a Carpet, which, although it is in the corner, is not called Carpet Corner. Jack learns that you have to sit on the Carpet and listen to the Teacher. Jack learns her name almost immediately. But it is not important because if you want to say something to her you have to Put Your Hand Up. (Mummy wasn't so right about that bit.)

At dinner time, which is actually lunchtime, they eat school dinners. Jack learns that he has to walk and carry a tray at the *same time*. He also learns that you have to choose between fruit or pudding. And that before you can have it, you must eat your plate *all up*. Jack has never eaten a plate before. He decides to skip dessert.

On Tuesday they start learning to read. He looks at the letter O. 'O, O, O' he says.

On Wednesday he falls over and bangs his knee. Somebody takes him to The Medical. Jack learns that it is nice there and he will get a Well Done sticker if he cries loud enough.

On Thursday he goes into the Hall for assembly. He

listens and he says a prayer and he wonders how long this will go on.

On Friday some of the bigger kids start calling him Tiny. He doesn't mind because the girls amongst them say he is cute. They pick him up and swing him round and round. He quite likes it in fact.

Starting School Again

On the first day, Mummy is shown her son's Classroom. She says a polite Thank You to the Teacher, and then takes the hint to leave. She reminds herself not to worry and that everyone will take a while.

In the Playground there is a huddle of mummies, a couple of forlorn daddies and the odd au pair. And a normal-looking one, too. Some she already knows, some she doesn't. Some of them look a bit scary. There is Jo and Hannah and Adrian and Catherine and Saskia and Duncan and Vincci and Justice and Lowri and Paul and Sonia and more. She wonders how she will ever know all their names.

On Tuesday she starts learning some names of the teachers too. She feels like she is ten again, calling everyone Mr this and Miss that. She looks around still confused. 'Who, who, who?' she says.

On Wednesday a Nit Letter comes home. She feels like crying when she looks at the tiny nit comb and her son's unruly mop. She feels worse still when she realises her own scalp is feeling a bit itchy.

On Thursday everyone is extraordinarily, unbelievably tired. She drops her son off and says a prayer. She wonders how long it will go on.

On Friday she goes for a coffee after drop-off with her friend Avril and their trio of pre-school boys. She doesn't mind that Sid knocks over the sugar bowl and that Billy leaves half of his drink. All in all, the week has gone quite well. And she realises she quite likes it in fact.

It is a hot summer's day at the end of July. School's out. We're snatching a break in Cambridge, staying in my parents' house while they are away visiting my brother, his wife and their little boy in Italy.

We've decided to go to the huge open-air paddling pool on Lamma's Land. It is free, enormous fun and guaranteed to wear the kids out a treat. Plus there's the added bonus of suggesting they look out for furry Alpaca-type beasts. In truth, we are probably pronouncing the name of the place all wrong to local ears, and the only hairy find we're likely to happen upon is the odd discarded sticky lolly. Still, it keeps us amused.

We arrive early. The boys strip to their smalls. A splattering of sun cream and they're in. There's a handful of other kids here already. Everyone's letting off steam. My lads notice a lone boy, between Jack and Billy in age. He has a trophy inflatable boat. They make straight for him, Sid tottering round the edge in hot pursuit.

The day passes in a blur of Piz Buin, shrieking, and the occasional pit stop for race-against-the-heat dripping lolly-licking competitions. The boys are having the time of their life. They hardly need our intervention. We get to watch languorously from the sidelines, our nostrils filled with that peculiar damp, paddling-pool smell that you get no other place.

And then it is time for the other lad to leave. His dad is calling him in. He knows his time is up and goes obediently to heel. Allows his dad to get him dressed. And then tears impulsively back to the knot of frolicking bodies that is our sons. Jack is pretending to fall over backwards, shouting stagey 'whoa's as he crashes into the water. Billy is splashing in circles round him, stomping up the spray with aplomb. Behind him he drags Sid in another inflatable boat, where he sits clapping and chuckling uproariously, a tubby, near-naked and thoroughly delighted little emperor.

Their new friend shouts to them from the edge, waving frantically: 'Got to go now! Came to say goodbye!'

Jack, catching sight of him, splashes immediately over followed by the rest of the cavalcade. I can't hear what they are saying. But I can see Jack extend his flawless young arm, and he actually shakes hands. The other boys clamour round and wave as their friend, responding to his dad's persistent shouts, finally turns heel and slopes off. His shoulders are round, his feet are dragging and he looks completely and utterly crestfallen. My boys meanwhile turn around and throw themselves back into the fray. With buckets this time. And lots and lots of flying water.

And then before we know it, it is late. We need to round them up, clap towels around their water-wrinkled bodies and get them home for tea before it is them that's melting down. So we give them the five-minute warning. And then the two-minute warning. And then Dirk shouts: 'Who's going to get to the towel first?'

And they all shout back 'Me!' 'Me!' and 'I do!', and as they belt over in our direction and we envelop their warm little bodies with our arms, I feel proud and sad at the same time. I rub the towel around the delectably chubby thighs of my damp and sun-bleached youngest, and I know that my carefree, freckled children are quite simply perfect. They are irresistible. And not, it seems, only to me.

Dirk is pulling a T-shirt off over the top of Billy's head. I admire the curve of his cheek, his impossibly long eyelashes and the fine line of his eyebrows for which I would need wax and good money to achieve on my own aged brow.

I am sad because I realise that this can only last for such a brief time. Everything changes. If only I had really made the most of it. My babies are already boys who are developing their independent selves. They already need us less and less. Our own friends are moving away, looking for a better quality of life outside London. Avril and Mark and the kids are off to New Zealand. I think back to the 'what next' conversation with Mum, and I reckon I need to start thinking about what I'll be doing next. Work? Not just yet. What then? Further education? Further babies? No. Not just yet.

I feel like the emperor in his new clothes. I didn't care much for normal rulerly trappings. Didn't want the career, the title, the money. I wanted instead to clothe myself with my children. Keep them wrapped exquisitely close to me. And so I did, and I have. Worn them close to my heart through thick and thin that is. But I need to keep my wits about me. Those swindlers Time and Age are lurking, ready to drape me with their fabrics. When the time comes, I must not act the fool and go on regardless, refusing to see the truth. There will be a point when I need to let go. Let the children move on. Develop their own social selves. Get on with their lives and resume my own.

'Now, who wants to run to the car?'

And we all bolt off. Except Sid, who stumbles, falls, and then outstretches his arms to be carried. Not just yet, I reflect with relief.

I am in the kitchen, loading ketchuppy plates into the dishwasher. Jack is colouring *and* staying in the lines. Billy is galumphing around my ankles, singing 'Robin Hood' at the top of his voice, pinging imaginary arrows from our home-made bow. The real sticks we'd picked up in the park had failed to twang correctly. Shame. Sid is lying on the floor wailing: 'Booky. Booky. I want *ru*. Read. Me. Booky!' He is not, I think, talking about Russell Brand's autobiography.

Unswayed by the fact that I have eyes only for the dirty melamine, he repeats the request again and again. And again. I like to think that I am the boss in this relationship but he's got his negotiating skills down to a T. Eventually I crumble and he gets what he wants.

Which is for me to sit down and pore with him over the visual feast that is Richard Scarry's *Cars and Trucks and Things That Go*. He has good taste. The book is legendary. Only I've already looked at it twenty times this morning, and the family of pigs are starting to ingrain themselves on my retinas. I feel like I am stuck in one of those optical-illusion science experiments. Any moment now I will see an old lady where a moment ago I saw a young one. Oh no, I'm getting confused. That is not an experiment. That is just looking in the mirror.

'Find Gold Bug!' he insists, nodding his head vigorously, his eyes scanning the page as he does so. Gold Bug is the small boggle-eyed flea who, not surprisingly, is gold. He is also to be found lurking somewhere sneaky and part-hidden in the depths of every page. My eager offspring never tire of seeking him out, knowing he is there, somewhere, amongst the cast of neatly clothed animals busily at work and play, and the dazzling array of 'real' vehicles like the pickle truck, the apple van and the toothbrush car giving hot chase to a toothpaste tube on wheels. It is a book featuring everything imaginable that moves. And it also has the uncanny knack of keeping my lot sitting still for entire minutes at a time.

I am thinking, I would like to find my Gold Bug too. Eventually. Then I sit at the table and pull Sid snugly onto my lap. I open the book and put on my imaginary blinkers that make as though I have not ever seen this page before, and I say, 'Now, where *is* that Gold Bug?'

Billy crowds in at my shoulder. He surely knows. Doesn't he? But if he does, he's not letting on. He is transfixed by the bedlam that is unfolding on the page in front of us. His face is a picture of wonder itself.

I return to the book and my finger traces out the squashed and spillaging banana truck, the upturned fresh-eggs van, and the exploding yellow mustard-tube lorry. There's a hose-squirting fire engine, a bubbling liquid detergent pick-up, and a whipped-cream three-wheeler whose pressurised canisters are firing randomly into the sky like a host of unchecked fireworks. A forlorn-looking mouse is standing aghast on his upturned car, a pastry-chef is losing all his flour, and a maple-syrup tanker seeps its sticky load, slowly south, downwards like a blanket of lava towards a log-jammed chinaware van. And look. There he is. Gold Bug. Inside. The china's a bit broken but everything is, obedient to the arrows, the right way up. It is all utterly and totally bonkers. It is a vision of my life.

'What a to-do!' I laugh, hamming it up.

'Don't worry. Mistress Mouse is there. She'll sort them out,' piles in Jack, felt tip aloft, unable to resist wandering over for a quick gander.

'Find Gold Bug!' instructs Sid.

And I do. And as I place my finger on the bog-eyed little critter in the midst of all this mayhem, I know that there is nowhere else I'd rather be.

My partners in crime are hanging on my every word. They are watching to check I don't skip a page or lose concentration midway through. They are like OFSTED whipping boys, observing that the teacher is going correctly through the motions. Am I outstanding, good, inadequate or downright pants at leading them through their lesson? Am I enthusiastic enough? Do I do enough silly voices? Am I spending long enough on it before fobbing them off again for the dishwasher?

The pigs get to the end of their journey, I close the back cover, and declare it 'the best book I've read all day!'

'Yay!' they chorus. I think I am getting a big fat tick in the 'good' box. And it does indeed feel good.

I am no longer a mum in her thirties who is rapidly getting older and sometimes feels like she's losing her marbles. Sometimes treading on them too. I am a spot-on teacher and I spread happiness around like melted butter.

'Again. Again!' instructs Sid, and I wonder if maybe I'm not *that* spot on after all.

Mummy County Primary School - Reception Class

Pupil report: Charlotte Moerman (aged thirty-something and a bit)

Charlotte has been on the Early-Learning Years Curriculum for a little while now. Overall, I am delighted to report that she is doing quite well, really.

Charlotte has made excellent progress in learning how to take her own coat off. She can usually do it within twenty minutes of arriving back home after unbuttoning everyone else's jackets, shoes and 'Why didn't you bring the car' tantrums after walking home from school.

Charlotte can do quite a lot of new things, mostly by herself now, actually.

Charlotte is particularly good at creative dance and movement. She smiles from start to finish. Even on the days when she forgets her kit and has to do it in pants and vest. She is very good at that. Smiling regardless.

Charlotte, though prone to daydreaming, is making a concerted effort to *concentrate*. She is shrugging off the cumulative build-up of pregnancy brain and is doing her level best not to forget all the important things while her head overloads with 'Hand over your mouth's and 'Stop hitting your brother's and 'Will you *please* put your shoes on for the fifth time of asking's.

Charlotte no longer wets herself when Daddy leaves for work.

Charlotte is able to express herself with control and confidence, really quite a lot of the time. Even when the finger-painting bonanza left the kitchen walls looking like the Sistine Chapel. She was spectacularly effective at demonstrating just how cross she was. In imaginative language too.

Charlotte has a secure knowledge of numbers zero to ten, especially in reverse order when counting down to the naughty step.

Charlotte's attitude has come on a long way since the start. She no longer drops her pencil deliberately on the floor just *because*. Even when certain others, naming no names, e.g., Dirk Moerman, are *still* at the office, in a plane, or going through a tunnel. Which happens to be in a pub.

Charlotte has learned to stop pinching things from her classmates. Like their voices when she is sick of the sound of her own, endlessly repeating 'Eat your carrots', 'Pick up your pants' and 'Aim for *inside* the toilet bowl just for a change, will you?'

May we wish every luck to Charlotte as she moves to the Not-*so*-Early-but-Still-Quite-Wet-Behind-the-Ears Years Curriculum. She will almost certainly need all the luck she can get.

And as I get to the multi-vehicle pile-up page *again* I read the words of Pa Pig in my best Pa Pig funny voice, and say: 'Well, we are almost home now.' 'Thank goodness,' says Ma.

And then I realise I am. I'm home. Thank goodness.

Epilogue

It is February again. We are in an Arctic rented hall. It's Dirk, the boys and me, plus my parents who've come along to help. Rain is pelting on the corrugated iron roof and radiators are hissing reluctantly into action. I prop up another line of triangle sandwiches on a suspiciously damp-feeling paper plate.

It is Billy's birthday party. He is having his first 'big one', as the expectation has now been laid. Jack expects the party. Billy toes the line. Sid, meanwhile, forages in the quiet corners for discarded drawing pins, Blu-Tack and popped balloon ends.

Failing any of those, there are sure to be sandwiches falling from the sky if he hangs around long enough. Because the sandwiches, I know for a fact, will not be eaten by the young guests. They will all be cheerfully ignored. I know this, but I still cannot help myself. I rise to the unwritten Mummy Rule of Hosting Kids' Parties that states 'To offset the sugar, fizz and E-number bonanza, thou shalt provide a couple of plates of sandwiches, some crunchy carrot sticks and perhaps a bowl of grapes'.

The kids, of course, will do what they always do anyway and pass over all these in favour of the cocktail sausages, the fairy-cake icing (the licked-off remains of the cakes themselves will be returned to the plate) and the European Hula Hoop

Mountain which seems to wash up at our door on occasions such as these. Not that the Hula Hoops tend to go south with any urgency. As anyone knows, they are chiefly provided so that every child in the room can slip one on each finger, wiggle their hands about, and consider themselves the cleverest wag in town.

I pop the plate of sandwiches on the windowsill in the absence of any free worktop space, and promptly spirit them off again when I notice the window isn't watertight and the bread is getting rained on. Mum is trying to hunt down the matches, last seen pretending to be a needle, shortly before disappearing into a haystack. Dirk is trying to crank up the radiator in the still-icy room saying 'I've tried but it won't go up any more!' Dad is whipping up the big boys who are whooping round the hall like a gang of angry natives on Coke. Sid seems to have lost his trousers. Everyone is hyped to the max, the entertainer still hasn't shown, and another balloon goes bang.

Billy had wanted a horsey cake. Adamantly. (There's a joke about a mounted highway man in there somewhere.) He had seen the model he wanted me to reproduce in my *Woman's Weekly* Kids' Party Cakes book. He hadn't wanted Gary the Ghost, Francois ze Frog or even the admittedly tempting-sounding Princess Shazza. None of these would do. What he wanted – exactly – was the Pony Club cake with two small plastic dollies on horseback in a paddock encircled by Cadbury's Chocolate Fingers.

'That looks lovely Billy,' I'd crooned. 'I'm just not sure we've got any dollies *quite* like that though. Do you think I could ...'

'No. I want it like *that*.' His brows had begun to knit but then he'd quickly changed tactic with a cock-headed enchanting 'please' that had me eating perimeter-fence chocolate fingers out of his little hand.

I had subsequently done my best to find a comparable pair of dolly-mounted toy nags. The fact that in the end I could fit only *one* of my equine finds on top of the smallish cake, and that it also happened to be riderless, was, I thought, a small point that could surely be overlooked. I'd congratulated myself on what I thought was the perfect cake. Just what the doctor ordered. A beacon of sugary hope that perhaps the party would go just fine. That I would *not* get stressed and end up run ragged. Like I do at every party. Something I tend conveniently to forget almost immediately after each one, selectively editing out the bad bits in favour of the good. Not unlike labour in fact.

At least this time the cake looks good, I think, as I dab at the soggy sandwiches with a kitchen towel. It is, even though I say so myself, a culinary work of art. There's the Cadbury's Finger perimeter fence, a Curly Wurly jump, green desiccated coconut grass, 'Happy Birthday Billy' icing and our all-important plastic pony popped jauntily on top. Perfect.

Only not in Billy's eyes it's not. He does not agree that a lone riderless horse is *almost* like two mounted ones. He does not agree that the improvised jump with number '3' flags on each fencepost is quite a good idea actually. He does not agree that the cake is, as I had thought, perfect. You can lead a boy to his horse cake, it seems, but you can't make him think it's up to scratch.

And so in protest, while I'm busy running round doing the last important little jobs like locating the vanished matches, he quietly sets about improving it. He gets hold of the lonely pony and takes it for a clip-clop round the field. Before anyone notices, the paddock becomes a hoof-cratered quagmire, the icing writing is in tatters, and the pile of artfully arranged toasted coconut 'hay' is now scattered around willy-nilly, looking disconcertingly like trails of strewn manure. Never has a more authentic pony paddock been created.

I take it surprisingly calmly I think. Not. 'Who left it in his reach? How can I fix it now? I can't *believe* it!'

And then I stop and listen to myself. I am the grown-up here; he is the child – the birthday child at that. I sound like a petulant teenager or worse. A sports star behaving badly?

I realise in a moment of truth that I'm the one smelling distinctly not of roses. I've been so busy dancing to my own requirements that I've overlooked Billy's spec. He wanted it one way; I delivered something else. So he's trying to modify it to his liking. It's his birthday cake and yet I'm still interfering, wanting to do it my way. Wanting to meet some mythical target when in fact the only aim is and should be to have a happy Billy at the end of it all.

I take myself in hand, remove the cake to a higher surface (though not the windowsill) to avoid the risk of the pony imploding his own paddock at least, and then turn around to smile at the first smattering of guests who are walking in through the door.

Then I take a step back as Billy throws himself into it. Let him be. It's his party and he can cry the shots if he wants to.

And he does and he has a ball. So, therefore, do I.

Later. It is nearly over. Everyone's exhausted, but it *has* been fun.

I've tipped the virtually untouched but decidedly sad-looking sandwiches into a black bin liner, and collected anything that looks unlicked and/or vaguely palatable for later (i.e., not much), and I've got the party bags in a battalion by the door, slices of the deconstructed pony cake nestling within. Mum is wiping down the trestle tables with a J Cloth. Dad was last seen wowing the crowds joining in 'If You're Happy and You Know

It', though he appears at some point to have disappeared for a quiet sit-down.

Which is what I fancy doing. Sitting down. Though not quietly of course. After running around like a headless chicken most of the day, I figure I can enjoy a quick breather and watch the last five minutes of our expensive but worth-every-crowd-controlling-penny entertainer.

Dirk is sitting with Sid on his lap. Most of the other kids are up at the front getting up close and personal with a probably spittle-damp microphone, delivering varying-ability karaoke renditions of 'Twinkle Twinkle'. Jack's already been up. He's keen. He'll be on *X Factor* 2020, if it's still going. Which it probably will be. Billy's less mad for the limelight. He's content just to watch. Which is what he's doing at this moment. Bunched up on the floor with his dad and his brothers, observing.

'Shift up a bit,' I say and plonk myself down with them.

I realise almost immediately I've sat on something squidgy. Maybe spilled jelly. Maybe a discarded sandwich. I realise I'm also not bothered and wink at the birthday boy who in turn rewards me with a 'love you' raspberry. Which is, I think, just the ticket.